Mr. Magoo Is My Role Model

Mr. Magoo Is My Role Model

Roy M. Mendelsohn

iUniverse, Inc.
New York Lincoln Shanghai

Mr. Magoo Is My Role Model

iUniverse books may be ordered through booksellers or by contacting:

iUniverse
2021 Pine Lake Road, Suite 100
Lincoln, NE 68512
www.iuniverse.com
1-800-Authors (1-800-288-4677)

ISBN-13: 978-0-595-35717-8 (pbk)
ISBN-13: 978-0-595-80195-4 (ebk)
ISBN-10: 0-595-35717-2 (pbk)
ISBN-10: 0-595-80195-1 (ebk)

Printed in the United States of America

Contents

Preface

September 11th. is a day noone can forget. For me it stirred the coals from deep within to write this book. I have written a number of books, each of them trying to communicate what I felt was important. However, I was always dissatisfied and knew something was missing. Until now I did not have a clear idea as to what that might be. This is the first book I truly enjoyed writing and it contains the missing ingredient..... Me!

I hope you enjoy reading it.

INTRODUCTION

I had just finished my last appointment late on a Friday afternoon. Driving home my mind was filled with questions and reactions to another week of coming in contact with new ways of looking at myself as well as others. Shaking my head in amazement, at how much there was to learn, my thoughts turned to my Zadie (Yiddish for grandfather).

Many years earlier he had acquainted me with the enormity of that undertaking which he considered a life long task. I found myself smiling as I recalled our walk together clear across the city of Chicago. It was very early in the morning of what was scheduled to be my Bar Mitzvah. He wanted to make sure I understood the full meaning of what I was about to do, even mentioning that he wanted to be there to support me in the event that it was something I didn't want to do. I don't think that he had any doubt that I would say yes, and had I decided not to I'm sure he would have been very disappointed. Yet at the same time I knew, as well as I knew my own name, that he was sincere. At that time he was the only person I felt comfortable enough with to be totally honest regardless of how it affected anybody, including him. In addition he was always true to his word.

When I was very young he used to hold me in his arms; the sound of his singing and the rhythm of his dancing letting me know how much he enjoyed my company. I felt so safe, and in some wordless fashion, like much more of a person. Later he told me many stories of incidents he had encountered and of how he had handled them. He ended each one with the same words like the chorus of a song "It was the honest way of living". Often I joined him in chanting these words. We both loved it. For example, he was a carpenter and used his skills to buy old, run-down buildings, fixed them up, and then sell them. Before they could be sold a variety of inspectors would come by to give their approval. Before doing so their hands were held out waiting for the expected payoff that was customary in that graft-ridden city. He would have none of it, making his position very clear. Subsequently, he would be faced with every nit-picking defect that could be found to turn him down. These were also accompanied by veiled, or not so veiled, threats. His attitude was that he was being given a chance to really discover what it took to be impeccable. Thus his buildings came to be known for that quality. He had no trouble selling them whenever they had reached a point where they could not be turned down, because......"It was the honest way of living".

So there he was explaining to me, at the age of thirteen, what it actually meant to become a man. It was not simply an empty ritual. In his words, the sins of my parents would now be my own. This signified that I alone was accountable for every aspect of my behavior. It took me awhile to grasp, but when I did, I shook my head in wonderment at what it would require of me to always accept responsibility for everything I did. This was the day of my Bar Mitzvah and I didn't see how I could ever accomplish it, much less before we arrived at the Synagogue. This really cracked him up and he couldn't stop laughing as he tried to explain that it would be a life long process. As was his style he then chided me for being in a hurry, while emphasizing how a dedication to, and love of, the truth and honesty could lead the way. This made sense to me as he well knew, for he had always encouraged me to follow my heart in everything I did. He stressed the importance of not being swayed by others' opinions, or by any other temptation for that matter. He had often teased me about my tendency to think too much with my head, though he would add that there was hope for me for I was aware such thinking only led me in circles. When we approached my destination he gave me a hug, stating that he just knew I had it in me to become what he called "a mensch". He hoped that all of the decisions in my life would be guided by my being true to myself.

I wondered why these reminiscences were popping into my head. At first I thought it must be because I was so deeply engaged in seeking the truth about myself. This approach was part and parcel of the career I had chosen, which was turning out to be everything I had imagined and more. Then suddenly it hit me. I had a weekend in front of me with nothing scheduled and the next night was the first Seder of Passover. This had been a very special event for me over the years, which highlighted the attachment I felt to my Zadie. He had been struck by the ravages of what would now be called Alzheimers disease, so that his ability to function, or even recognize who people were, was declining rapidly. As I got out of the car to greet my two young children it struck me that they would never really know him as I did, nor would he get to know them. However there still was a spark of life left in him, at least whenever he saw me, and I suddenly felt a strong urge to see him before he died. On a number of occasions, although he hardly recognized anything or anyone around him, he always knew when I was near by. I would tell him that now it was my turn to tease him about losing all of his marbles, and he would playfully poke me in the ribs admonishing me for making fun of an old man.

At dinner that Friday night I mentioned the pull I felt to attend the Seder, which must have been contagious, for it also appealed to my wife. My daughters, age three and one and a half, responding to our enthusiasm, clearly approached it like we were off on an exciting adventure. Although it involved driving six hundred miles all night Friday, getting a little sleep before the Seder Saturday night, and then turning right around to drive six-hundred more miles on Sunday, it was well worth the trip. The entire extended family was there, pleased and excited to see all of us, and my Zadie came to life probably for the last time before he died not too long afterward. My oldest daughter still remembers the event, especially the place he occupied.

In some ways for him it was a return to the past. Just as it had been during our growing-up years my cousin (four years older) was on one side, while I was on the other, both of us propped up on pillows. We teased and joked with him as he went through the ceremony, exaggerating our usual efforts to make him go faster when he slowed down or slower when he quickened the pace. He, in turn, feigned irritation or took a moment to call attention to the meaning of a given ritual. The tears welling up in his eyes (and in ours), as he would reach over to give first one and then the other a big hug, said it all. Here we were two grown men and an aged, senile grandfather, touching each other deeply by recreating an interaction that kept the child in all of us alive.

Looking back I can see that it was this quality in him that was the source of what I thought of as wisdom. He had words that just seemed so right. During my growing up years, for example, I just loved the idea of Christmas. The concept of honoring the love we felt for others, and expressing it through the giving of gifts, struck a positive chord in me. The holiday ritual of decorating a tree also seemed like a joyous experience. It was hard for me to understand the negative reactions I received whenever I mentioned such things to many members of my family. It was as though it was somehow sacriligious for a Jewish person to celebrate the birthday of Jesus Christ. Thus the first Christmas after establishing my own family a Christmas tree was included, which did not sit well with my parents. In great anguish (and knowing the strength of my attachment), it was suggested that it would kill my grandfather. Because of my curiousity I did introduce it to him and his response possessed the essence of what I consider to be wisdom. He listened and, when I had finished describing what it meant to me, commented on how very lucky I was. When he saw a Christmas tree he was reminded of pogroms, where everyones life and loved ones were in great danger. He still momentarily shrunk back at the sight. Then with his characteristic warm smile he put his arm around me and expressed his pleasure that I could see something joyous.

I have now lived long enough to become a grandfather. Meaningful experiences with my grandchildren have brought with them a new and surprising revelation. Earlier I had only thought of what my grandfather brought to me, with no conception of what I may have contributed. I can now see I was as much a giver as a receiver, and it explained to me one of the reasons I felt so effective when I was with him. The bond we formed lives on within me as a source of strength and vision when I am faced with hardship or darkness. It also makes me aware of the wordless wisdom I possessed as a child.

Wisdom refers to the power of judging correctly what is accurate, and being able to tell the difference between what is true and false. Unfortunately this admirable human trait is usually not recognized unless it is expressed in words, and even then not until the words can be understood. We are used to thinking of wisdom as a rare commodity, which can only develop slowly as a consequence of facing and mastering a host of sometimes harsh and difficult life experiences. The implication is that it requires a wealth of information and knowledge, as well as perspective and sensitivity. Therefore, it would seem almost incomprehensible for a child to have achieved such a remarkable attribute. Yet we are continually given at least small glimpses of evidence that children do have that quality. How often have we heard a child make a profound comment, clearly indicating some essential truth in a few simple words. The expression "out of the mouths of babes", reflects a universal awareness of this ability in children. Along with it, however, is an implied element of surprise as though it is an unexpected occurrence.

A child's incisive and penetrating perception of what is genuine or false, of what is straight forward or distorted, in most instances exist as vague impressions susceptible to being over powered and defeated by adult logic. Children need help in finding the right words, which then resonate with these impressions, giving them substance and meaning. When important people in a child's life do not grant validity to their perceptions, either disregarding them or worse seeing them as dangerous and prohibitive, children tend to feel doubtful both about the experience and about themselves. A child's wisdom is a present offered to loved and needed persons, just as the proper words to express it are a present given to a child. The exchange enhances both.

The story of The Emperor's New Clothes portrays the destructive influences of exploitation, greed, and intimidation. It also shows how the voice of a child can expose fear driven distortions by making a clear statement of the truth. Thus what is surprising is not that children have access to this kind of vision, for their growth and development depend on it, but that there are instances when they can articulate it so well. Nothing is more nourishing to children's growth than to find caring adults receptive to their input. A child must be heard in order to be seen.

What goes around comes around, and I have travelled from being a child whose grandfather brought him a gift of words to becoming a grandfather wanting to carry that message to others. This book tells the story of my education.

Cindy

Walking toward the conference room, after spending the morning getting oriented to my ward assignment on my first day in psychiatric training, I felt wonderful. It was a very hot day so I took off my tie to be a little cooler, while popping a stick of gum in my mouth. I was looking forward to my first meeting with the head of psychiatry, a famous and highly respected psychiatrist. Little did I know what I was soon to be confronted with, since I had unwittingly chosen two pet peeves of what turned out to be an extremely brilliant, knowledgeable, but irascible man. I took a seat near the front of a large room, gradually filling up, for we were all there to hear him talk about a wide range of topics in what he called a colloquium. The room became quiet as he began by welcoming all of the new residents in the audience. Scanning the room his eyes glanced at me for a brief moment and he launched into a diatribe against wearing casual clothes without a tie when engaged in professional activities. I didn't disagree with anything he was saying, I.only wondered why he was so incensed. When he shifted to stating that there was only one thing worse he could think of, and that was chewing gum, I realized he was referring to me. Now he focused his attention directly towards me and asked if I could explain why I did not have a tie on, and also why I would be chewing gum. I felt very embarrassed, but also angry that he would make such snap judgements and treat me in such an insensitive way in front of so many others. So it was that I answered his question with all the sarcasm that I could muster, "because I didn't have a bathing suit that would match my tie on this hot day, and the gum was an insurance policy to keep me occupied if I got bored".

What a first impression for me to make, but there it was and I wasn't in the least bit sorry. As time went on I did come to admire him for his teaching and organizational skills, yet as a person I did not care for him at all. On another occasion, again in a colloquium, he made an active appeal to his audience to please tell him why noone came to talk with him. He wanted to offer anyone the opportunity to speak with him about whatever they might have concerns or questions about. A number of people made comments to the effect that he was such a busy man they did not want to bother him. He recognized the falsity of these

1

comments, brushed them all aside, and continued to emphasize how much he wanted to hear the truth. Against my better judgement, for I didn't believe for one second that he had any interest in hearing the truth, I stood up to speak. I told him that I personally had no desire to talk to him, because it seemed to me he only wanted to hear what pleased him. Furthermore if it didn't his harumphs would close off any further discussion. In characteristic style he then harumphed a few times and changed the subject. An interesting sidelight to me is his choice of the word Colloquium for these meetings. They were conversational in their content, which is the root meaning of the word colloquial. However, Colloquium is defined as the portion of a complaint in a lawsuit for slander, which alleges the speaking of the words which constitute the offense, and connects them with the plaintiff. It appears as if he unconsciously(or perhaps consciously)chose the right word. He certainly conducted himself as if he was entitled to slander others, or to bait them into returning the favor. In that context there is no doubt that I responded to his invitation.

Imagine my surprise when I received a personal invitation to be part of a week long study to investigate murderers. This would be followed by a series of mock trials, wherein the most competent lawyers would demonstrate their skills by destroying the validity of psychiatric testimony. I had been selected by the head of psychiatry as one of four psychiatrists who would participate. I agreed and it turned out to be an incredible learning experience in regard to testifying in a courtroom. The lawyers were impressive in their ability to hone in on any evidence of uncertainty, ambiguity, intimidation, or waffling, and then use it to shred any semblance of credibility. They brought out clearly how the law is strictly a chess game, having nothing to do with the truth, justice, fairness, or any other idealized attribute. However, they also showed how vital it was in testifying to be absolutely truthful, for even the slightest deviance is pounced upon to totally decimate the rest. Now it became apparent to me why I was chosen. Although I was awkward at first, I was able to duel effectively with the lawyers. He had seen this quality in me and knew the lawyers could use it to better demonstrate how to function and get a point across under these circumstances. Over the years I have had occasion to testify in court a number of times and the lessons I learned during that week were invaluable.

A lawyer, who had heard me testify in a case where extremely abusive parents were deprived of child custody rights, called me to ask if I could possibly evaluate a very young child. There was some urgency involved, since he feared the child would be removed from a loving foster home soon; unless the judge could be convinced that it was contraindicated. I agreed and so it was that I met Cindy.

She was a twenty month old bundle of energy who burst into my office with her foster parents trailing behind. She immediately showed me a stuffed animal she was carrying and directed me to hold it. I did so but obviously in a way that made her dissatisfied, as she kept moving it around until it met her exact specifications. She was then openly delighted and with a sigh of relief plunked herself down on the floor right at my feet. Her foster parents observed all of this looking somewhat uncomfortable and started towards getting her to sit in a chair. I simply remarked that I would like to hear their story, but at the moment it looked like Cindy was telling me something and I wanted to make sure I understood. With that I said to her I thought she was informing me that she, like the stuffed animal, knew exactly how she needed to be held. More importantly she wanted to make sure that I would listen to her and try to make it happen. Her head snapped around as she gave me a huge smile that lit up the whole room.

Originally I had planned to meet with Cindy's foster parents to get some idea of the quality of their relationship with her, followed by my seeing Cindy at a later time alone. They had decided to bring her when they had trouble finding a babysitter, and figured they could take turns being with her in the waiting room. They also hoped I might want to see them all together and that option would be available. In the background was their worry about the passage of time. The foster parents were explaining all of this, as Cindy occupied herself by exploring every object she could reach. Periodically she brought one over to me eager to get an explanation as to what it was. Each time I answered her factually at first, and added a simple statement to let her know what I had been hearing from, and saying to, her foster parents. She clearly loved being included in this fashion.

How much she understood, or how well I was grasping the meaning of her behavior was as yet unclear. Nevertheless it looked like there was a good start in that direction. Her foster parents described what she was like when she came to be under their care at three months of age: pale, thin, poor appetite, cried very little, and no smiles; quite a different picture from the child she is now. They revelled in watching her gradually come to life and as she did winning their hearts. Her birth mother had been heavily involved in drugs and though abuse was suspected, there was no concrete evidence to support it. The only thing known was that Cindy was seriously neglected, and at times abandoned for significant stretches of time, due to the mother's drug induced behavior. She was then placed in the foster home and the mother disappeared. Over time the foster parent's attachment to Cindy deepened, which led to their initiating adoption procedures.

In the midst of their taking this step the mother suddenly emerged upon the scene, proclaiming herself to be free of drugs and demanding her parental rights. The foster parents anxiety concerning the time factor centered upon a court action that was scheduled to take place in just a few weeks. They were afraid Cindy would be removed from their home, perhaps even forcibly, and the trauma they anticipated her having to endure just broke their hearts. It was accentuated by Cindy's reaction to being with her biological mother. There were three meetings ; two with the foster mother accompanying her, and one alone. In the first one Cindy was herself, much in the manner she had greeted me. In the second she was shy, refusing to leave her foster mother's lap. She returned from the third very upset: clung to her foster mother for several days unable to leave her side, and had great difficulty sleeping at night. The foster parents believed that Cindy somehow sensed what was happening, though they had not as yet talked to her about it. They knew it would be important for her to be included, but because of her young age they were at a loss as to what to say or even how to say it.

I then spent two sessions alone with Cindy. She was eager to come, readily left her foster mother to enter my office, and was more verbal than I had expected from our previous encounter. She had brought her stuffed animal, but this time wanted me to speak to it. "Talk to safonie"(I found out later this was stephanie;her favorite object named after an older cousin). I followed her direction by telling her why I was seeing Cindy. While I was talking Cindy interrupted periodically to either add something, ask something, or react to what I was saying. When she spoke it was somewhat hard to understand all of her words., but she did manage to get across her meaning. I explained that she had two mothers; one who carried her inside until she was big enough to be born, and the other who took over to help her grow up. Cindy listened intently to this and pointed to her belly button to tell me this was where she had been connected to her mommy. I asked if she knew which one. She shook her head no with a puzzled expression. I then told her that the woman she had been seeing was the one. She stopped me in the middle to make a face; "scared me" as she scrunched her shoulders together. "Where's mommy?", she said going towards the door. I simply stated that she was quite right that was her mommy, even though it was her second one. Again she stopped me, "will you get my mommy?". "Yes", I said, deciding at that moment that I would in fact do everything I could to make it possible. When I informed her of my decision, she came back to my chair; "some more" were the words she said quite clearly.

I took her words to mean that she wanted me to continue explaining. Therefore I told her there were lots of big people in the world who thought she should go back to her first mommy. "Oh-no-no", as a frightened look came across her face. Continuing I said that I wanted to be her voice and let them all know how awful that would be for her, and how they just had to make sure it would not happen. "Tell safonie", she whispered. I did so, emphasizing how big people often could not believe how much children knew about what was best, and even worse didn't take what children did know seriously.. When I informed Stephanie that I was going to speak for Cindy, she had Stephanie give me a big hug. There was now no question in my mind as to whether she was old enough to grasp the meaning of my meeting with her, and of my role in the upcoming custody trial.

I arrived at the courtroom a few minutes late due to unusually heavy traffic, so I had no idea as to what had already taken place. Cindy, her foster parents and lawyer were sitting on one side of a long table; her biological mother and lawyer were on the other. All of them looked up at me as I entered. The only thing I noticed was a worried frown on both foster parents faces(later I discovered that the judge had just explained to them the significance of parental rights law, and the various things that would have to be proven in order to have these rights terminated.). I was immediately asked to testify. After being sworn in, the attorney representing Cindy's foster parents simply asked for my findings. It took me about twenty minutes to describe the nature of my contact, what took place, and how I understood its meaning. He then requested that I repeat my recommendations and the basis for them. I then placed great emphasis upon my feeling of certainty that Cindy's foster parents were now firmly established in her mind as her parents. Furthermore they had done an excellent job in helping her to overcome the trauma associated with her biological mother. It appeared to me that the parental rights of her foster parents needed to be protected, in order to be in Cindy's best interests.

Slowly the opposing lawyer approached me and in an overly polite manner asked a few questions about my credentials. He then asked if I had seen Cindy's biological mother. My negative answer obviously pleased him, triggering a barrage of questions to which I gave brief replies. "How can you make a judgement about her without seeing her?". I can't", I replied. "Did you not recommend that her current foster parents retain custody and even be allowed to adopt this child?". "I did!". "What evidence do you have then that giving the mother custody would not be in the child's best interest?". "She told me!". "Do you want us to believe that a twenty month old child is first of all capable of conveying that information and second that it would in any way be reliable?". "Yes". "Doctor, how can you make such pronouncements and assume they have any validity?".

Now it was my turn. I spoke at length about the factors that were known and their significance in the development of a young child; the obvious trauma of her early months and the role it played in her failure to thrive. Elaborating on the concept of the cure determining the cause, I outlined her response to the parenting she was now receiving. I indicated that it was understandable to me that it might appear strange to base so much on the validity of such a young childs feelings, not to mention how they could even be communicated with any degree of clarity. Just as I was beginning to explain in some depth how I came to my conclusions, the mothers lawyer interrupted stating something to the effect that the court did not require a lecture on child psychology. Precisely at that moment, probably reacting to the emotional tension rising within me(and most likely in others also), Cindy broke loose from her foster mother's arms . She ran straight to where I was sitting and jumped up on my lap. Clutching her stuffed animal to her chest, her voice rang out loudly, "doca keep talkin!".

Everyone was stunned, but most importantly her proclamation made a huge impact upon the judge. He immediately put an end to the court proceedings and spent the next two hours meeting separately with the mother, the foster parents, and even for a short time alone with Cindy. The foster parents were informed the next day that they had been granted full custody and that they could go ahead with their plans for adoption. There were even arrangements made whereby the biological mother could be included in Cindy's life if she so desired, though the foster parents would be in the position of deciding just when and under what conditions.

It was an amazing experience for me; not that she needed a voice such as mine to allow hers to be heard. I knew that from the beginning. Sad but true, children's voices, especially young ones, are rarely listened to or given credibility. The striking part was how much I needed the exclamation point provided by her words for my voice to be heard. Here I must have come forth with thousands of words and the outcome was still hanging in the balance. She introduced only three to settle the matter.

George

I couldn't have found a better setting for my psychiatric training than the one I chose, except for one small detail that I hadn't even considered. The $2,000/year stipend just wasn't enough to support a family. Searching for a solution I signed up for a governmental five year program, which paid a liveable income in return for spending two years in an outlying hospital. So it was that after two years of training I went off to an understaffed facility, after which I would return to complete my residency. It didn't feel like a sacrifice to me, since I thought it would be a good opportunity to consolidate and put into practice what I had been learning.

Unbeknownst to me the hospital I was assigned to had prepared for my arrival by placing over 200 patients, and a small staff of nurses and aides, in a separate building. This was to be my area of responsibility. I found out later that they had crefully selected what they considered to be their most troublesome or problematic patients. In addition they placed their most difficult employees to serve as the clinical staff. This was really quite ironic, for the criteria as to what constituted a good patient and a good staff person was defined by how readily they conformed and followed orders without any kind of protest. It turned out to be a marvelous choice. If I had spent the entire two years evaluating patients to determine who was strongly motivated to find help, and select a staff of people who were most dedicated to providing help, I could not have done as good a job.

Nevertheless when I first entered that building the changes had just been completed, everyone was new to each other, and absolute chaos reigned. I will never forget that first day. Here I was twenty eight years old(and looking much younger), I had no idea of how to begin or even what to do, and I was to supervise and/or provide meaningful psychiatric care to more than 200 extremely disturbed people. I would have some help; there was one RN and anywhere from ten to fifteen aides per shift with fewer at night. Several things were clear to me immediately, which I firmly stated to everyone I spoke to(both staff and patients). I needed time to get to know them all as well as I could, I would not be making any decisions until I had some semblance of understanding, and I was quite new to this whole process. After a few tests here and there from patients with me answering no to any requests, and encouraging staff members to proceed as they usually did, everything gradually settled down.

Now I was faced with the serious dilemma of how to bring some kind of treatment, under these difficult circumstances, with my limited knowledge. The way I thought about it at first was that it would be impossible, if for no other reason than the numbers. How in the world could I treat such extreme illness in 200 people? I wasn't even sure of how to work with one. Even by including the nurses and aides I couldn't see anything that made any sense. Then it hit me. What if I reversed the numbers? what if the patients provided the treatment, and perhaps also at least participated in running the wards(there were four of fifty patients each)? Then the staff could serve them as consultants or supervisors. I had no idea whether it could work or not, but at least the numbers were more reasonable.

Convincing the staff that what I had in mind was in any way feasible was an enormous undertaking. I knew that without their active acceptance of the idea, and willingness to set aside all they were accustomed to doing, there would be no point in proceeding. Fortunately this was a really dedicated group of people. They had been very dissatisfied with the way things were done, and made no bones about it(which was why they were assigned to this building). In addition I could tell that they were becoming more trusting of my motives. They saw me struggling to find real answers to the daily problems that arose, appreciated my efforts to be available at all times, and it was a new experience for them to have a doctor value their input. At any rate they slowly began to become enthusiastic and we decided to see how it unfolded as it was introduced to the patients.

Initially it looked like it would be a complete failure. I held daily meetings with the patients, explaining what I had in mind and why, while encouraging them to add their opinions. The response I received was either blank stares or an occasional outburst of some delusional idea. My bubble of excitement burst, but then it dawned on me to listen closely to the few things that were said. Delusional though they might be, and a reflection of their psychotic illness, there was a theme to all of the utterances. They were expressing their feeling of total helplessness and crying out for some kind of guidance or direction. So I shifted my position and instead presented the way we were now going to run the wards.

A committee composed of eight patients would be formed, whose function was to determine what the best way was to conduct how the ward was run. This group would have the authority to decide upon any issue whatsoever that affected a given individual, or the group as a whole. This would include everything that was possible to provide, as well as their daily activities. The staff would be available to carry out their decisions, or to serve as consultants if they were uncertain about anything. On the other hand, if anyone had a request of any kind it had to be presented to the committee in person, so that questions could be asked in order to gain the information necessary to make meaningful decisions. There will be daily sessions, during which these matters can be brought up.

Once I made this announcement, I asked for volunteers. I indicated that since we were instituting a new procedure I would make the initial choice, based upon whether I thought the person was able to handle the responsibility fairly. However, after the committee was established these decisions would also be theirs to make. A long silence followed. Much to my surprise a man stood up and with a deep scowl on his face began a condemning tirade against what he called a conspiracy. He continued on in this vein for a few minutes before launching into a series of challenging accusations directed to me. "Who do you think you are?! You can't give us permission to run this ward! You're just a young punk! What do you get out of this anyway?".

Thus it was that I was introduced to George. He had been a patient in the hospital for more than twenty years. Noone knew much about his background, nor was there much in his chart. It was a thick chart, however, filled with descriptions of violent episodes leading to a series of electric shock treatments(the treatment of choice for such matters I guess). At one point a lobotomy was being considered, and though there was nothing to specifically indicate why it was not done, from then on there were apparently no more outward expressions of violent behavior. Instead he was quite reclusive, constantly mumbling and grumbling to himself. Any attempts to get him to participate in anything were only met with a hostile "get outa here!". Early there were some references to his hearing voices, having delusional ideation, and being extremely paranoid.

I responded by treating what he said as deserving an answer. First I explained my reasons for trying this method, stressing my inability to see how adequate care could be given the way things were. I then said a few words about who I was, as well as outlining my level of training and experience. Finally I addressed his question as to what I got out of it as one I couldn't yet know. To my amazement he proceeded to grill me, in a challenging fashion, as to how I would manage a variety of problems in the form of "what if" questions. These ranged across a broad spectrum from people asking to go home, to wanting special supplies or equipment, to how activities would be handled. My response was to emphasize that every effort would be exerted to enable whatever the committee approved of. I couldn't guarantee it, only that I would try. It made me realize, and thus have a chance to say, that I should not have a vote for then it could easily slide into being a sham.

While this interchange was going on between us, I was struck by how adept he was at eliciting the truth or searching for defects and flaws in reasoning. An image crossed my mind of the potential he had to be a great chairman of the committee, which I then said aloud. Upon appointing him I suggested that he might want to take over the job of picking the other members. I was expecting my suggestion to fall flat, but without a moments hesitation he proceeded to take over; and take over he did. Not in any way did he go along with my approach, his style was markedly different. Turning toward a man huddled in a corner he emphatically demanded that he come forward; no further questions were asked . The person he had addressed just quietly got up, came to the front and sat down. In short order he selected the rest and the committee was established.

With each passing day the committee became more functional. The staff of nurses and aides got increasingly involved in the spirit of the undertaking, and everyone could see the positive effect that was emerging. After a period of testing by the committee, to see whether their decisions were honored, it became apparent that their authority was genuine. Although I had no vote they were eager for me to contribute my opinions. Especially in the beginning they would almost deliberately go against whatever I thought, which led to interesting dilemmas for me and somewhat risky situations for some of the patients. For example, during this early period of testing two of the patients put in a request for a weekend pass, which was granted after very little discussion. In my role as consultant I questioned the absence of seeking information, so that the necessary data would be available to make an informed decision. My words seemed to be ignored, though later on it turned out that they had been taken very seriously. The two patients travelled by bus to a big city where they presented themselves to authorities as having run away from the hospital. To their relief they were returned quickly. This incident had a big impact, for afterward the interviews became quite intense. Not only was my input sought, but it was apparent that many of the members were trying to learn what to look for.

It was an eye opener to experience how much insight and awareness this group of very sick and disturbed people had in relation to each other. When applied to themselves it was often non-existent, as the waves of their trouble washed over them wiping out any vestiges of perspective. George, in particular, was a superb interviewer. He was abrupt, to the point, and quick to recognize and discard what he considered to be nonsense. Thus on several occasions a patient would either ask or demand to go home, and George would almost shout in his characteristic style;"Are you nuts, all you do is goof off and talk to those stupid voices of yours! There's no way in Hell you could make it!". At other times he was thoughtful and for him compassionate, especially when the person looked both serious and vulnerable;"why don't you wait awhile? get your shit together, maybe put in for a visit and see how it goes!". The others on the committee slowly began to follow his lead, bringing out their own ideas into the discussion. On a few occasions, when the requests had to do with changing how the ward was run, there were arguments among the committee members. I became important then as they looked for me to serve as a referee. Everyone knew that I was the only one who had the authority to actually change a heretofore established policy, and it was very touching to see the variety of reactions when a change was instituted. The patients were at first shocked, but then strikingly cooperative. The nurses and aides were initially skeptical, and noting the difference in the patients attitudes, increasingly enthusiastic. One consequence was in the patients becoming involved in providing care and even handling some of the menial tasks.

The hospital had a procedure for dealing with administrative matters such as passes, visits, or major changes in hospital privileges. All wards were closed, but a given patient could have open door access if it was approved. When I had first arrived, I knew from the moment I entered that there was something amiss in the attitude towards patients in general. There posted on a bulletin board in the patients dayroom of every building was a highlighted notice, "Patients who are hallucinating will not be allowed in the canteen". I laughed when I saw it, since I thought the absurdity was hilarious. In that environment, however, none of the physicians could see why I considered it to be out of line. At any rate there was a weekly meeting of all the doctors, chaired by the hospital director, during which all requests were automatically granted or on occasion questioned. At this meeting I simply presented all of the committees recommendations with the implication that they were solely my own. They were accepted and approved with no questions or discussion. I was glad about that, for I had a feeling(later verified) that if what I was doing was known it would cause trouble.

A consultant to the hospital from a big city nearby met with me periodically, and he was intrigued when he heard what was happening. He sat in on one of the committee meetings, afterward shaking his head as if he couldn't believe what he had just witnessed. The remarkable way the committe functioned astounded him, and so he thought I ought to make a presentation to the staff of the entire hospital. I told him why I was reluctant to do so, but he was convinced it might be good for them to know. Subsequently he mentioned it to the director, who almost had a fit. He couldn't believe the things he had been approving of, and his anxiety increased the more that he remembered. After much discussion he hesitantly agreed to wait and see how things went.

At about this same time George placed a request in front of the committee to be given an overnight pass. In spite of the fact that he had not left the confines of the hospital for close to twenty years, everyone granted it without discussion. I wondered what had prompted his request, but it seemed so innocuous I also could see no reason to question him. So it was that he went out and proceeded to place calls trying to reach the president in order to complain bitterly about the way he was running the country. His calls were traced, so that the police picked him up and brought him back to the hospital. The director, upon being informed, became enraged. We had several discussions, during which I tried to emphasize the validity of his concerns in regard to the safety of a given patient. I also indicated my openness to receiving any input that suggested an element of danger. However, I expressed my opinion that I thought this situation was relatively harmless and was warranted in relation to its benefits. My attitude disturbed him a great deal, since he thought it showed a lack of concern for how the hospital was perceived by the community. Then, to my dismay, he started visiting the building in the evenings, when I wasn't there, causing a great deal of confusion by writing orders counter to the committees recommendations. When he totally ignored my efforts to speak with him about it, I did the only thing I could think of; I wrote an order refusing him admittance into the building. It was unfair to expect the nurses and aides to be able enforce it, so I did so myself. The consequence of this act resulted in my being called to Washington D.C. to present evidence justifying my stance(they ultimately promoted the director into an administrative position).

Meanwhile George once again requested a pass, but before the committee had time to act on it he asked to see me alone. I was struck by the difference in his attitude in this one-on-one meeting. In place of his usual gruff, cynical posture, he was awkward, reticent, and shy. He wanted to know if I intended to let him go on his pass if it was approved. I tried to explore why he was asking, since it implied that he might not want to go and he easily could just withdraw his request. It was obviously quite painful to him (and quite moving to me)to reveal how ashamed he felt of being frightened to leave the hospital grounds. What was even worse, however, was to face what he thought were the condemning looks of others if he never made a move in that direction. I told him that I supposed I could go against the committees decision, but wondered if that wouldn't elicit alot of anger in the others as well as himself. Pulling himself up in his chair. his old attitude returned(this time with a slight smile); "what's the matter Doc can't you take it?". I did turn it down, surprisingly noone complained, and business was carried on as though nothing unusual had occurred.

Without realizing it at the time, I was in the midst of learning an important lesson about labels. The experience with George captured the significant influence a label can have upon how a person is treated. As far as I can tell diagnostic labels never really fit any human being that I have ever known. Of course there is always some element of truth or accuracy in what they describe, but partial truths are in fact the most harmful of all(complete misrepresentations are easy to discard, whereas a degree of accuracy readily reenforces an erroneous view). What a difference it makes with a person like George, for example, to see him as a paranoid schizophrenic with delusional and aggressive tendencies, as a cantankerous curmudgeon witha cynical chip on his shoulder, or as a helpless, frightened, vulnerable little boy overwhelmed by the demands of a hostile world.

When I left the hospital, after my two years were over, I was excited at the prospect of returning to finish my training. My goodbyes to the people I had worked with were sad, but with George it was especially meaningful. We both knew he would in all likelihood spend his life in a hospital. Before I left he wanted me to know how grateful he was for being treated with respect. He knew that the circumstances within the hospital would change, but he would always treasure what it felt like to be regarded as a helpful person. I thought he was referring to what he had done on the committee that had been of such help to so many. Looking back I now realize how much his words apply to what he had done for me.

Eddie_____

There I was standing at the door fumbling around trying to open it, feeling a little frustrated until I looked down at the key I was using. This was my first day of residency in psychiatry. I'd gone through eight long years preparing for it and I could hardly believe the moment I had dreamed about was finally in front of me. How in theworld I had managed to get through pre-med, medical school, and internship I'll never know. Jumping through all the hoops that were required went so against everything I valued most. At last it was here and I thought I would burst with joy and excitement. So what was I doing trying to open the door to the ward I had been assigned to with my car keys. It was my first recognition that indeed there was such a thing as an unconscious, introducing me to that part of my being that was scared to death I had made a wrong choice.

When I was sixteen I had worked in a shoe store; pure torture for me, but it had cemented a resolve to never,never chose a career that I would want to retire from. At the time it was the only work I could find that didn't interfere with sports, which I guess made it tolerable. I pretty much thought I would move into something involving my interest in atheletics;a teacher or coach, Ididn't know what. The only thing that had meaning to me in one way or another involved either chasing, hitting, or catching one kind of ball or another.

It was about one year later that I decided what I wanted to do with my life;in a sudden moment that actually caught me by surprise. For years whenever I was asked why or how I chose psychiatry, or becoming a doctor, I always knew the answer. For a long time, however, I was too enbarrassed to say. I gave the usual replies of wanting to help people, of being interested in the body and its functions, or of my curiosity concerning health and disease. Of course these things had some truth in them,but they were not the reason I picked medicine and psychiatry in particular as my life's work. The real answer came to me in a flash when I saw a movie that dealt with a psychiatrist trying to get at the deeper truths that tortured a troubled patient. My reaction was one of a loud "click" inside—That's what I wanted to do! I had no idea as to what a psychiatrist was, or more importantly what I had to do in order to become one. Upon looking it up and discovering it meant being a physician, I recall thinking "Oh no! I'm going to have to go to medical school "as I realized how long it would take. Little did I know then that it would be more than time that gave me trouble.

Dealing with what I have come to call "misauthorities" was very difficult : at times i'm not exactly sure for which party. Certainly I made things more troublesome for some (which I must admit was often fun for me). However, the opposite also took place; where I was the one who suffered (Isuspect with the other getting a degree of pleasure at my discomfort). During my years in college and medical school I had numerous encounters that made me wonder why I continued on such a path. I saw so many incidents of injustice, insensitivity, and outright deceptiveness, many of which were given noble names. Although I was frequently outraged by all of this, fortunately they were balanced by enough experiences of integrity and a love of the truth that I continued on toward reaching my goal.

The experience I had with my car keys emphasized to me that I was surely not immune to self deception. At the same time it also brought to my attention just how essential it was for me to follow my heart in whatever I did. The phrase it's easier said than done comes to mind, but i'd have to say that it seems like the opposite is true(at least for me).Whenever my heart is not in something i've done it has been incredibly hard. I do not think I could have gotten through college or medical school otherwise, and my internship year without a doubt would have simply been impossible.

Looking back, I still don't see how I managed. First I was overwhelmed by the nature and size of the task, compounded by the expectation that I was in any way prepared for what was required. In the hospital Ihad chosen the intern was in charge of the emergency room(the very reason that I had selected it). I knew in my choice of psychiatry it would be unlikely for me to keep sufficiently informed in other branches of medicine to have any degree of competence. Yet it was important for me to possess the knowledge and skills necessary for handling life threatening situations, at the very least to recognize what could or couldn't be done in an emergency. In one way it was a great choice, for I did meet every conceivable emergency. In another it was horrible. The hospital was poorly staffed and I was expected to take care of situations that were way beyond my capabilities. I did the best I could and before the year was up I even had a small measure of confidence.

It was an eye opener for me, however, to discover that there were many doctors who simply did not seem to care.When I was on call it was my responsiblity to be in charge of the emergency room, and there was always an attending doctor whose job it was to back me up if I needed help. Especially in the beginning this was quite often(I can readily understand how they might not exactly have been thrilled upon receiving a call from me),but many did everything possible to avoid appearing in person. Fortunately I had the authority to insist. Once these people saw that it was easier to respond to my calls than to have me insisting they show up even for a skinned knee the problem disappeared. I was then confronted with a much more serious matter. It was hard to determine with a few of the attending doctors, particularly the ones who had arrogant attitudes, whether it was an expression of supreme confidence in what was required or a way of covering up an underlying sense of their inadequacy and helplessness.

Happily my residency in psychiatry turned out to be everything I had hoped for. The entire ambience of the setting communicated a devotion towards seeking out the truth. The genuineness of this undertaking was unmistakeable, as nothing was exempt from being explored including the setting itself. I could feel myself learning and growing and I knew I was in the right place. The initial years primarily dealt with adults, and as my training shifted to focusing primarily on children what I considered a strange phenomena emerged. It was as though any sensitivity to,or understanding of, the children I was seeing completely disappeared. I was at a loss to explain it, since from the outset this was what I was most drawn towards. In addition I was very aware that it was the child in adults with whom I made the most meaningful connections. I just couldn't figure out what was happening to me, but I knew something was wrong even though others were reassuring me that I was progressing very well.

I sought out a woman who I had noticed quietly sitting in on various conferences. She rarely spoke, seemingly listening as she knitted. However, when she did speak, her words penetrated right to the heart of whatever was being discussed. I told her in great detail every thing I could recall about my contact with the children, giving many examples of my interactions. Finally she stopped me and simply asked, "when are you going to enter the room?" My first reaction was of confusion as to what she meant, but then I realized she was referring to my somewhat stiff and formal attitude. The only thing I could say was that if I entered the room with a child I would be joking and teasing. I didn't see how that would be in any way professional. How could I be a doctor if I was so flippant about serious matters?(At the time I hadn't yet understood that play was almost always about serious matters,even though play isn't possible with a serious attitude). Once again she simply asked me another question, "What's the matter, are you afraid to discover your mistakes?" This question had a big impact on me. It enabled me to drop my facade, and I did indeed make many mistakes, but I also learned a great deal. More importantly my inability to establish emotional connections with the children dissolved.

It was at this point that I met Eddie. Ultimately he would provide me with the most penetrating, painful lesson about the value of the truth, and the horrible consequences of self deception, that I have ever received. It remains alive to this day(over 40 years later), serving as a constant guide and reminder to me. Right from the moment I saw him I was struck by his appearance, for I had never seen such an unremitting expression of anguish, accentuated by what could be thought of as bizarre behavior. Initially this 7 year old child did nothing else, during the time we spent together, but rock back and forth patting his cheek while loudly moaning as he did so. He was quite heavy, almost obese, and had to be led from place to place since he gave no indication whatsoever of any initiative or desire with the possible exception of satisfying his hunger both at and between meals. The depthof his suffering was constantly in evidence, though its source at this stage was totally obscure. His parents had brought him a long distance with the conscious intent of finding help, though it was quickly apparent that there powerful motive was to be free of the pain they felt in his presence.

The early sessions with him were experienced by me as a challenge;even though his behavior never varied. I tried everything I could think of in an effort to reach him, from questions, to impressions I had in regard to how tortured he looked, to the theories I had read concerning this kind of phenomena:all to no avail. After several months of daily contact with no indication that anything I did had the slightest effect, my reactions began to show my increasing frustration. At one point I even found myself half shouting at him,"Aren't you ever going to say anything?!" After this outburst I felt terrible, and again consulted with the wise woman I had spoken with earlier. My major question had to do with how long I should continue to try. When or how do I recognize that either I, or the child, or a combination of both of us, are just not what is needed? Her reply was quite short, "When you stop feeling anything either for or about him". I left her office extremely dissatisfied.

Something in that interchange must have affected my attitude, for to my amazement two days later Eddie spoke to me for the first time. On this momentous occasion it was obvious that he wanted to come to his appointment, since noone was either pushing or dragging him. He began by telling me what had taken place that morning. His speech was extremely rapid, as though he couldn't get the words out quickly enough. He began by revealing the reason for his peculiar behavior, especially the loud moaning sounds. There was a little man on his shoulder shouting obscenities into his ear. All of his effort was exerted in order to quiet this viciously condemning voice, which accused him of every imaginable crime ranging from murder, to the whole gamut of perversions, to incest. There had been no waking respite until that morning when the little man's words, though still attacking, were startlingly different to him. While he was telling me what the little man was saying it was my turn to be startled.. They were the precise words that I had used in those moments when I felt most frustrated. "Are you ever going to talk?, how long can this go on?, can't you say something?". It was a striking mement for both of us.

Everything changed, at first slowly, gathering momentum with each passing day. His appointments became the center of his life; a place to speak freely of whatever occupied his mind. During the early stages of this transformation all of his thoughts and feelings revolved around his current experiences. There was a highly driven quality in his voice that made the depth of his underlying anxiety apparent. Every example he gave of a given interaction, or of anything that happened to cross his mind, immediately unleashed a barrage of questions. "Was that wrong?, should I have done that?, Am I sick to feel that way?, how can I get well?"Often I either had no answer, or I might see something that led me to comment on what he could be feeling. My words usually reflected my search for the cause of his distress. At times I noticed how fearful he was of anything that could be construed as aggressive or angry; either within himself or in others. The most consistent theme that was in the background of almost all of his productions was a terrible fear of just being dropped or abandoned in some fashion.

Months now passed with Eddie widening his scope of involvements; he even initiated a move to enter a public school. More and more he wanted to be considered a "normal" 8 year old boy. He was quite frightened initially, but to his amazement he developed a friendship, found that he could actually learn and enjoy it, and wonder of wonders volunteered to participate in his school's band. A recital was scheduled and as the time approached he became increasingly panicked at the prospect of playing the drums in front of a large group of people. Somewhat haltingly he wondered if I could be there. In exploring what it would mean to him, he simply remarked that whenever he imagined me in the audience his fears quieted down. The night arrived with me sitting as close to the front as I was able to get. He caught my eye, we both smiled, and he proceeded to vigorously beat on the drums. It was another powerful moment between us and led to another shift in how he conducted himself.

His attention spontaneously turned to exploring his family relationships; a seemingly forbidden topic up to this point. He introduced the subject by indicating his acute awareness of its importance if he was to get better, but he just had been unable to do so. It felt much too dangerous. A sense of humor was beginning to show itself in his sessions, and now he laughed in trying to describe his mother. The best he could do was to draw me a picture. In struggling to get it just right he kept giggling, finally explaining the scribbled lines I was looking at. He couldn't decide whether to place himself inside of her as if she had swallowed him up, or the opposite to put her inside of him. Appearing puzzled for a moment, he silently nodded and stated that probably both were true. This made him think of his weight and wonder if he was fat because he had swallowed her, or if he was determined to get too heavy for her to take him in. There was no trouble at all in painting a picture of his father, as he put it there would be a blank page. He was always busy, away on business, or preparing to leave. His younger brother was now five years old and he imagined him ruling the household.

At this juncture two events having powerful emotional meaning for him entered his world. One concerned his parents who had been informed of the progress he was making and decided to visit. The other had to do with circumstances in my life, making it necessary for me to entertain the possibility of moving to another state. When his family arrived I was still uncertain as to when, where, or even if I was leaving. It became important, however, because now in his anxiety driven style he kept asking me if I'd be leaving him. This was occurring in the context of his feeling cut off from any emotional contact with the members of his family. For me it became confusing to know how to respond honestly. By this time it was abundantly clear to me that the absolute truth was essential, for anything less was devastating to him. When his anxiety was in no way relieved by any of my attempts to link it to the experience he was having with his family; he had openly felt like they were alien strangers eager to leave him so they could return to their own planet. I was then pretty sure that he was already sensing what was not yet definite, so I informed him of my dilemma. He eagerly questioned every detail until he was totally convinced that there was really nothing else I could do. His emphasis was on the importance of a child not being abandoned (the circumstance involved one of my children needing special care that was only to be found elsewhere). Meanwhile it did become necessary for me to be moving, giving us six months before it would happen.

Now his questions shifted to wondering if he could come with me. There was a different quality to his voice and his entire attitude. Deep down inside I knew it would be the right thing, at least to see if there was any way for it to be a viable possibility. The logistics of accomplishing such a move were mind boggling, and I can vividly recall how overwhelming they seemed at the time. Retrospectively it is clear as a bell, though in the moment the idea was filled with doubt and confusion. Nevertheless I did take it seriously, since I was unable to push it aside or treat it simply as a fantasy. Thus I consulted with a number of people. Their answers were all variations on the same theme. They perceived my desire to bring him with me as a reflection of rescue fantasies, most likely the residue of unresolved narcisstic injuries along with a resulting overidentification with this child's plight. In conjunction with whatever tendencies I had to be seen as a valiant hero saving a hurt child, they considered any step in such a direction was destined to be destructive to both the child as wellas myself. Their final point was that there were plenty of other good therapists who could pick up on the work that had thus far been done, and the entire setting was capable of providing the kind of support I would be unlikely to even come close to finding anywhere else. Some who I spoke with were quite adamant, strongly advising that I not get lost and stray from my primary task of helping him to address his abandonment anxiety and to say goodbye.

I listened, took it all in, and worked hard to convince myself of the validity of these observations. Yet, I still felt a nagging sensation that something wasn't right, for there was a background feeling of relief at being free of the responsibility. Strangely(looking back I do not think it is strange at all), I did not even think of consulting with the woman who had been helpful to me earlier, nor did I realize that I had neglected to consider her. This only serves to further underscore the extent of my self deception. How Eddie and I got through those last months is still painful to remember. He became increasingly withdrawn, while my efforts to "help" him understand the impact of his early experiences on this separation did very little.

My request to visit him periodically and write on a regular basis was emphatically denied by the setting as contraindicated. The consensus of the clinical staff was that it would interfere with his forming a new therapeutic relationship. Approximately five years later, out of the blue, I received a letter from the clinical director. During this period of time he had continued to withdraw, ultimately refusing to participate in anything, while spending all of his waking hours pacing back and forth. A decision had been made that he was basically unreachable and he was to be sent to a state hospital in his home state. Someone had remembered my interest in him and I was being notified in the event that I would like to visit.

I didn't know what to expect as I waited in the conference room where we were to meet. The door opened and he shuffled in dragging his feet, while the person who brought him quickly disappeared. He was much taller(a teenager now), sloppy in his dress, noticeably heavier, with scraggly unshaven facial hair. I could have cried ; he looked so forlorn and defeated. Pacing the room he didn't give the slightest indication of noticing my presence, nor did he react in any way to the words I spoke. The time I spent that day seemed like an eternity: I found out later it was two hours. At the outset I just talked; about why I had come, what I had realized about my mistake, what our relationship had meant to me, how much I had learned frpm him, and my deep sorrow for what he had to endure as a consequence of my blindness. After awhile I lapsed into silence. He continued to pace for a long time. Then from the far side of the room he stopped and turned toward me without looking at me. In a grunting voice(so different from the last time I heard him speak), he began to talk. "I know who you are". He went on to say that he let himself trust someone once, and he would never do it again. He had no interest in the reasons, he only knew that I knew what was the best and I turned my back and walked away. Clamping his mouth shut, he shuffled out the door and walkedaway. I guess it was his way of saying now it was his turn to do the same.

I believe that for Eddie the devastating factor was not that I hadn't taken him with me. It was the fact that I knew it was right to try, and then did nothing about it including not letting him know. Consequently I was not honest with myself, or him, about my inability or unwillingness to assume responsibility for his total care. In its place I put his anxiety as being the problem that had to be addressed, rather than my own reluctance to enter more fully into providing what he needed. The truth must always lead the way. Granted such a direction may not always be clear, or for that matter it may not always be possible to follow even when it is.

The memory of this experience has been alive in me ever since. Whenever I am tempted to stray it rises up within me to remind me of just how destructive self deception can be, and of how vital it is to search for, find, and be directed by whatever is right.

Sandy

Although I did not have words for it, I think I knew from a very young age that what is referred to as stress is caused more from lies and deception than from simply telling the truth. Therefore, when I applied for psychoanalytic training, it came as a surprise to me that one step in the process of approval was to participate in what they called a "stress" interview. The idea was to see how you handled anxiety arousing situations, by creating one in the interview. Psychoanalysis attracted me primarily because of its devotion to the truth, so it was hard for me to imagine just how they would create stress in the interview. I had heard from others that there was a policy to see people afterward to make sure they were not too disturbed to leave on their own. I figured they must have alot of people who lie apply for training and this was their way of weeding them out, but it didn't seem to fit with what I envisioned an analytic approach to be. Rather than being anxious or fearful when my turn came, I looked forward to it with a great deal of curiosity.

Entering a room with an empty chair at the front, facing a group of analysts, I realized that I did feel somewhat shy and uneasy(I'm not sure how many so I must have been more anxious than I was aware of). I immediately thought that this must be the stress they were referring to. After a pause I was asked a variety of personal questions and I could feel my discomfort dissolve as I answered. The questions became increasingly intimate in nature, expressed in an accusatory tone, with no time given for a thoughtful answer. At first I was taken aback by the insensitivity, but then it hit me. This is what this group of people considered to be stress. It struck me then as strange, not stressful, and just as suddenly as it began the questioning stopped. There was a long silence, during which I was reviewing my reactions to what had taken place.

An analyst sitting in the front row began to stare at me intently until he caught my eye and smiled. I'm not sure to this day exactly why, but I somewhat automatically smiled back. Now the grilling of me began in earnest. "What are you smiling at?. What were you thinking behind your smile?. Do you always smile like that?. they came at me fast and furious. After a few efforts to respond as honestly as I could, which were interrupted, I answered their questions in a way that they clearly did not expect. I was feeling a combination of disappointment and anger, so I told them precisely what I thought of their so-called stress interview. It was deceptive, dishonest, and manipulative in the worst way. If they wanted information why not seek it in a more straightforward manner—by asking! It seemed to me to be a very non-analytic approach to gathering information, not to mention the sadistic components that I was sure as analysts that they couldn't help but notice. If this was an example of how they thought and taught, it made me have second thoughts about being a part of it. I found out later that this was the last stress interview that they conducted, and I like to believe my words had something to do with it.

Nevertheless I found my psychoanalytic education to be invaluable from a number of perspectives. On the positive side it opened doors to my understanding of human development by providing treasured guiding principles. On the negative side it showed me how easy it was to confuse genuine truths with concepts, actions, or directions that sounded logical but had no substance. They may have simulated, resembled, or even corresponded with what was right or true without really being so; they were plausible not genuine. This was especially the case for me when it came to the definition of psychoanalytic treatment itself. So much emphasis was placed on distinguishing it from psychotherapy, as though anything that did not follow certain rigid rules was somehow either suspect, deficient, or a poor substitute. The idea that a couch, or a specified frequency of meetings, was essential as a condition of the treatment never seemed right to me. I could see where it might be the case if it came from the patient, but to have it imposed in my view went against everything psychoanalysis stood for. When it came to treating children the situation was reversed. Here to use the couch, for example, was thought of as contraindicated. A variety of reasons were given to explain why this was so, mostly centering around a child's supposed inability to handle the force of the resulting regression.

In the midst of my struggle to gain a deeper understanding of what appeared to be contradictory ideas, I was also following the requirements necessary to complete my training. A significant element revolved around clinical work. In my case, since I wanted to be a child analyst, I needed to have three adults and three children in supervised treatment. The adults were relatively easy to find, but to gain credit I had to be seeing three children at least four or five times per week. Furthermore the children had to meet specific criteria for them to be acceptable, which essentially meant they had to have a "neurotic illness". The idea was that the demands of "psychoanalysis proper" were too great otherwise. I had managed to find two children who had been approved; though one was thought to be "too sick" and I had received special permission to see the other only three times per week. It was at this stage that Sandy entered my life.

The initial contact was an urgent phone call from Sandy's father who was very worried about his eleven year old son. He felt something had to be done and soon. Both parents had been trying for a long time to get him to see a doctor, but he had adamantly refused. Thus, I saw his parents first to discuss what they could do. They both went into detail describing Sandy as a very troubled child almost from the moment he was born; fretful and colicky as an infant, poor appetite and problems sleeping all of his life, morose and withdrawn as a toddler, always unhappy. Separations were difficult, school has been a constant struggle in that he obsesses over homework, and he has no friends. Every aspect of his life seems to be painful. They have tried to get him to see a psychiatrist or psychologist since he was five years old, but his refusal to go is so extreme they kept hoping things would change. The puzzling thing to them is that he never at any time indicated that he did not want or need help. In fact, he frequently will express a wish that someone could help him. Recently he began saying that he had no desire to live, which frightened them and so they called. I listened and then suggested that they not leave the decision up to him in anyway. Instead simply inform him that they had contacted a child psychiatrist and let him know the time of his appointment. The next day I received a call from his father to let me know how right I was. They had left my office, told him precisely what I had said, and were then shocked when he readily agreed. More than that, he looked almost eager to go.

The moment I introduced myself to Sandy I could see that something was wrong. I had approached him in the waiting room where he sat reading a magazine, but as soon as I mentioned my name his face fell as though the end of the world had just arrived. When I asked him about his reaction, he became hesitant, looked embarrassed, and quickly changed the subject. Pointing to the couch, he wanted to know all about it. "Why is it here?". I referred to it as a place someone could be able to speak more easily of their thoughts and feelings without being distracted, adding that it could also be a trampoline. He smiled, "can I use it?". Which way?, I asked. With that he literally ran and pounced onto the couch. Much to my surprise, for I expected him to use the couch as a trampoline, he lay flat on his back and began to talk rapidly. More than that, for the remainder of our therapeutic contact(about five years), he never varied from lying on the couch the entire time. Occasionally he shifted his posture slightly, but for the most part he remained in a supine position after commenting how safe it made him feel to not move.

Initially he wanted me to know why he felt so disappointed. For as long as he could remember he has wanted to see a doctor. He knew there was something very bad affecting him inside, but no matter how hard he tried he felt totally helpless in being able to stop it or even to ease the pain it caused him. His parents have been on his back to get help, yet they didn't seem to grasp what he also found hard to put into words. He was so terrified of every adult he has ever known, or for that matter any adult period, that it was too scary to imagine himself talking about his trouble to one. With each passing year the problems and his despair kept increasing. Then to his great delight, his parents told him the other day that they had made an appointment for him with a child psychiatrist. He could hardly believe his ears. Recalling a magazine article he had read about a twelve year old boy graduating from college, he immediately assumed his parents had at last found a child he could come to for help. Laughing, I commented how I could readily see why he had felt so let down.

The next day he couldn't wait to tell me about a dream in which he had been riding on a magic carpet. It swooped up and down and he had to grip it tightly so he didn't fall off. There was more to the dream, though he could only recall going through dark clouds, brief moments of sunshine when he could see a city below, and of becoming alternately excited and scared. This led to our talking about dreams in general and what they might reveal if we could understand their special language. He was intrigued with the idea . Glancing down at a small section of the couch that was repaired with black tape(the couch was made of black vinyl), he casually remarked that the carpet in the dream had a spot on it just like the one on the couch. He saw the connection right away, stating that he must be pretty scared of his own thoughts referring to the ominous quality of the dark clouds in the dream.

This beginning period gave every indication that Sandy could make use of psychotherapeutic help. He was certainly suffering from turbulent, as yet unidentified emotional difficulties, and possessed the kind of psychological mindedness and motivation that would be important in finding solutions. In addition, I had to admit he appeared to be an absolutely ideal candidate for my final requirement. Not only did he clearly express his wish to meet frequently(every day was what he thought would be best), but he also had spontaneously chosen both the couch and a supine position as the safest most useful way for him to proceed. My supervisor was astounded, as was I, for supposedly children are not amenable to such an approach.

It was not long before the other shoe dropped. Gradually, as Sandy's treatment became a part of his daily routine he was allowing the full extent of his disturbance to emerge. His life was a nightmare for him, almost literally. He kept seeing threatening figures out of the corner of his eye, which disappeared as soon as he turned in order to get a better look. In his words he was extremely paranoid, and just knew that someone was trying to invade his body. It could not be anything except the devil. He becme obsessed with wondering why he was the target. The only thing he knew for sure was that it had something to do with his possessing some hidden secrets. Although he was unsure as to what these might be, the only relief he ever feels is in those brief moments when his bladder is completely empty. Thus it was that he felt compelled to urinate at the slightest hint of pressure, making his day difficult. Nighttime was even worse. Each time he was falling asleep he had to double check, which made sleep almost impossible.

My efforts to interpret the meaning of these symptoms were at times welcome and led to his elaborating further. Thus my comments reflecting on the figures menacing him as aspects of himself opened up avenues to powerful feelings that were frightening to him. For example, at one point he imagined a dirty, slimy cab driver trying to creep up on him. When I wondered if it reminded him of anything in himself, it immediately triggered a memory of being fascinated with his bowel movements and playing with them. At another point he thought of a horned devil, very evil and scary. This brought up the rage and resentment he often felt toward two younger brothers. With great emphasis and even glee, he wished he could chop their heads off. When I suggested his preoccupation with his bladder might have more to do with some emerging sexual feelings, and even some masturbatory activities, he became more upset. Meanwhile he was showing signs of increasing distress, as well as becoming more openly hostile and aggressive.

The depth and extent of his regression concerned my supervisor alot, raising questions in his mind as to Sandy's suitability for a psychoanalytic process. I, in turn, was worried but only as to whether I was on the right track with him. I thought that I was, though I also had many doubts. The question as to whether it was, or was not, a so-called psychoanalytic process seemed totally irrelevant. I was advised to see him sitting up, not allowing him to use the couch, and to consider less frequent appointments. At this juncture I was informed by the Psychoanalytic Institute that I had been selected to present a case to a world renowned analyst who was coming to visit. It was to take place in front of a large group and they hoped I would accept their invitation. I thought about it alot, for I wasn't sure how comfortable I would feel under those conditions. Finally I agreed, thinking it would be a great opportunity to get her input on my conduct with Sandy.

The big day arrived and there I was facing a little pixie of a woman with a foreign accent in front of at least one hundred people(most of them analysts). I liked her immediately. She just had the appearance of someone to whom you truly could say anything. Once she asked me to begin, I started to talk and my awareness of the audience practically dissolved. Quite respectfully she stopped me to inquire if there was a reason that I wasn't presenting process notes. She had seen the packet of notes on my lap and wondered why I hadn't opened them. I knew why and only hesitated a second before deciding to just tell her straight out how I felt. I told her that I was worried about the patient I had selected to present; he brought up questions that seemed to be contradictory to many psychoanalytic ideas concerning treatment and children. Therefore I wanted to present him in the most accurate way that I could, which was to tell it not read it. I added that I had noticed whenever I wrote process notes, without fully realizing it, there was a tendency to edit so as to present a prettier picture. She smiled and nodded, signalling me to go on. When I had finished describing Sandy as best I could, as well as the way I participated with him, she spoke at length in general terms about the problems in treating such a child. There was then a series of questions and comments from the audience, most of them critical at the idea of exposing such a fragile child to the rigors of a psychoanalytic process. Although she agreed, she also added that it was important to not be so rigid in our thinking. She thought there was much to suggest that this child was making use of the experience in a positive way, and it was too early to be so definitive. With that she turned to me and stated, "Dr. Mendelsohn, you are a courageous man".

Although these words may have been meant as a compliment, I certainly didn't in any way feel courageous with Sandy. If anything I felt confused, uncertain, lost at times, worried, and occasionally reassured by what seemed like validating responses from him. Thus I said, "I think you mean I may be using poor judgement". She giggled, nodded her head vigorously, closed the meeting, and offered me the chance to discuss it with her in private. There she thanked me for being so direct and honest with her; it was true, but she hadn't wanted to embarrass me in front of a group. She proceeded then to outline what she really thought. For me it was a wonderful experience . Just getting to know her in this way, and to see how she took in information to understand someone, opened doors for me to gain more clarity not only with Sandy but also with others.

She pointed out several things to me, some in the form of questions and some as direct statements. The questions revolved around what she considered to be a central focus of any treatment. Where was I in the child's mind at any given moment?(not necessarily directly or explicitly but reflected in how he interacted).

She noted a tendency in me to overlook brief moments of irritation on his part that quickly passed and were never questioned or spoken about. This might be an area that held a key as to his secrets. In addition he very seldom mentioned his parents, at least not directly. My focus on the peripheral vision images as parts of himself she felt was helpful, but incomplete. They could also represent aspects of parental figures, and thus a ready receptacle for buried secrets. Finally she underscored a moment she felt had been a determining factor in his engagement with me. It was when he ran to the couch and I asked him how he intended to use it, implying that it was all right for it to be a trampoline. "What a powerful message to let him know that you were receptive to anything that he might bring in, and so he did, only not quite what you expected". Overall, in her opinion, Sandy was not the usual kind of child we think of as being able to use psychoanalytic treatment. Nevertheless it did appear to be a worthy venture, and she ended by encouraging me to be even more playful.

I followed that advice, and in becoming more openly playful, I realized how much I had been affected by the depth of his disturbance. He, in turn was less at the mercy of his paranoid self attacks. This resulted in his connecting them to the disturbing feelings associated with an abandoning mother and a demanding, potentially violent father. Sandy's grim, serious, paranoid attitude dissipated, and in its place a wry, sarcastic sense of humor emerged. Instead of aggressive outbursts he now had a sense of enjoyment in exposing hidden truths in others, and could appreciate the value of finding them in himself. Previously where he would retreat in despair if his thoughts, feelings, or wishes were ignored, now he was pleased that he could see the reasons why it had occurred. Earlier he erupted angrily to his siblings taunts, whereas now he found creative retorts that were fun to deliver. Growth and integration became the order of the day. We completed our work together with Sandy feeling proud of his accomplishment. He was also finishing high school and looking forward to a time when he could help others. Laughingly he stated that he would be the child they might be searching for.

Sandy began by looking for a child who would also be able to treat him. Instead he found someone to treat him who was also able to be a child. On the other hand I was looking for a child who had the "strengths" necessary to be treated "psychoanalytically". Instead I found someone who could use the strengths of psychoanalytic treatment to truly become a child. It turned out to be a good match, since we both learned an important lesson. Sandy was right he did need someone who could understand what it meant to be a child. However, a child would be very unlikely to have the necessary strengths. I was also right, in that psychoanalytic treatment does nourish and foster the necessary strengths to be adequately treated. However, the whole purpose of treatment is to develop those strengths. It would be highly unlikely to need treatment if they were already present.

Gangs

When I was applying for psychoanalytic training, several interviewers were genuinely curious as to why someone with my background would be drawn toward this profession. They were referring to the emphasis on intellectual functioning; upon thinking rather than doing, and upon silent reflection in place of action and discharge. My answer was immediate, though I did not have the exact words to explain what I meant to myself much less to someone else. I said that as a child I climbed trees. The interviewers already knew about my history of what they thought of as "acting out" behavior; little concern about obeying rules(more accurately no concern about rules that made no sense), truancy from school(through high school I never attended a full day. In fact I could not use a real note, since I had a friend sign all of the forms on the day I entered), membership in a gang that was always in some kind of trouble, and involvement in athletics to the exclusion of any other interest. Under todays standards I am sure I would have been thought of as having an attention deficit disorder. What they did not know was another side of me that I usually kept quite private. Climbing trees captured it completely. In that silent arena, away from the world of others, I could contemplate what was most vital and important to me. Surrounded by the comforting support of something alive and solid(the tree), I could allow my private thoughts and feelings to rise up and fill my being. Although I didn't really think of it this way at the time, I was truly getting acquainted with who I was. Looking back I can see that I was extremely idealistic, constantly struggling to discover truths about myself and others, and to following moral principles and values in spite of all appearances to the contrary.

My moral values have evolved over time, shaped by a host of experiences and relationships. It has been fascinating for me to note the ones that have been influential, for on the surface they seem to be so disparate. The most powerful by far was provided by a beloved grandfather, for whom integrity, honesty, a love of the truth, and seeing with your heart were the only path to follow. Upon that foundation, of all things, it has been my participation in a number of what I will call gangs that my guidelines have developed. Some possessed values that I loved, some that I hated, and some a mixture of both.

My first contact with what I would consider a gang was at the age of six. I had just moved into a new neighborhood, having been accustomed to engaging primarily in solitary pursuits(riding a scooter, exploring the area, throwing a ball against a wall, etc). Upon stepping out into this new world I was immediately accosted by a group of children; some my age, some a little older. They were in no way friendly, and several went out of their way to block my path. I felt quite intimidated, retreating back into the apartment building I now lived in. Each time I ventured out this group would suddenly appear. It finally dawned upon me that unless I was willing to remain a prisoner I had to confront the situation, and so I did. I was awkward at first(I had never been in a fight before), but amazingly to me once the fight began my fear dissolved. What took its place was an intense feeling of anger, which was expressed in my not holding back whatever strength a slight, skinny six year old child can possess. Lo and behold everything changed. Instead of hostility I was asked questions like, "how fast can you run?", :what's your name?", "do you want to race?", where do you live?". Without my knowing it this was my initiation into the gang and I had passed their test. In the process of doing so, I had learned alot. First in regard to myself; that being intimidated makes you a prisoner (a victim of your own fears), while asserting yourself, though it may open doors to excesses of feeling, it also gives substance to your dignity. Then in regard to the gang: the unspoken recognition even at this early age that a group is only as strong as its weakest link. What a revelation. They ganged together in order to feel safe, but before they could open their ranks to any newcomer they had to know that the qualities they valued were strongly honored.

Looking back it seems strange to think of this group as a gang. We certainly did not think of ourselves that way at the time, and even more never considered that what we did was guided by moral principles. Had anything like that been mentioned I'm sure we would all have laughed at the idea. We were just a bunch of kids doing our thing in response to whatever came our way. Thus, for example, there was a yard we cut through as a shortcut to school. The woman whose property it was became furious everytime we passed, screaming at us to get off of her grass. She then put up a sign warning us of dire consequences if we were to walk on her grass. To us the answer was simple. We just dug up her grass so that there was none to walk on, while we continued to use the shortcut. In our view we had obeyed her sign, at the same time sending her a clear message as to how we felt about being treated that way. The morality of the group was such that had she made a request we would have gladly complied. The dictionary defines a gang as a number of persons associated together in some way or as a group of children or youths from the same neighborhood banded together for social reasons. Thus we were indeed a gang. Morality is defined as relating to, serving to teach, or in accordance with the principles of right or wrong. Here, also, we were united in a number of beliefs as to what was right or wrong, and what we did reflected those beliefs.

Each passing year brought more challenges and opportunities to develop and express our beliefs, though it always was shown in some common spontaneous action. Never was any thought, much less discussion, given to whether we were right or wrong. For example, noone had any money, yet occasions arose where the baseball we had been using got totally unravelled. There was never a question as to what to do. A trip was required to a local Woolworth's 5 and 10 cent store to slip a baseball into a long sleeved shirt or a pocket and then off to the ballfield. We wouldn't think of visiting a smallstore with an independent owner; that was merely wrong because he had to make a living. A strange morality in some ways, but it did not feel as though we were doing something wrong. Of course we knew it was stealing. However, Woolworth's would not miss it and we would have our ballgame

Another example centered around Halloween. For our group it was a time to cast off all restraints in finding creative ways to cause havoc in the lives of those who may have given us a hard time during the year. We had passed through the usual things like soaping windows(and waxing them once we saw the owners using it as an opportunity to wash them), sticking pins in doorbells, removing lightbulbs in hallways, and generally being a nuissance. At the age of eleven we decided it was time for something that would leave an unforgettable impression. A large apartment complex, anticipating trouble(for good reason, since they had chastized us often in response to a number of complaints from the residents)posted a guard at the front to prevent such things as sticking pins in doorbells and attaching various objects to the windows. This left the back stairways accessible to us where we could gather garbage cans and lift them up on the roof. From there it was a small step to remove a screen from inside a number of chimneys(this was my contribution as I was the only one small enough to reach them). The final element was to empty the garbage cans into the chimneys. The garbage was then deposited directly through a fireplace into the living rooms of the apartments. It was great fun in the planning and execution, but the ending was spoiled somewhat when the police caught us climbing down. Retrospectively that may have been the most significant part of the experience, though I would not have considered it as such then. We were taken to the station where we were bawled out, with many implications as to the possible punishments we would have to endure(the most serious probably having our parents notified). After what seemed like an eternity the police simply let us leave, and I now can see probably got a kick out of it. The entire experience, especially the ending, served to strengthen the bond that held us together. I have to admit that I loved the morality of that gang.

At the age of twelve I moved again, supposedly to have more opportunities to meet others of the same religious background(I had been the only jewish child in an Irish catholic community). In short order I came in contact with, and an integral part of, what was even labelled a gang. The initiation process was familiar, though not identified as such. It occurred on a snowy fall day, as I stood staring into space after school in front of the building I had just moved into. Three boys from my new classroom wandered by throwing a football. Recognizing me they asked if I'd like to join them. I was pleased and we had a two against two tackle football game, with no equipment, which was the roughest game I'd ever been in. They were surprised, because of my small size and appearance, by the aggressive way I played(they told me later they had expected to send me home crying and were kind of disappointed at the outcome). At any rate I was then invited to participate in a larger game the next day with the entire group; adding that of course I'd have to cut school to get there on time. This was a first for me; I had never missed school before without a legitimate reason. Although I did feel somewhat uneasy I was also excited, as I knew I had just been accepted by a group that I sensed would take me to new levels in challenging authorities(I should say misauthorities). My assessment turned out to be right beyond anything I had anticipated. Parts of it I liked alot, especially in the beginning, but over the next four or five years it reached a point where I was no longer comfortable with it.

Most of our activities together centered around a variety of sports, depending on the season, and I just loved the unspoken principles on how a game was played. Team play was a number one priority, period. If anyone on the team(or in the group)was treated unfairly, there was no doubt about the response. The perpetrator was now the target of retaliation from all of us. The same principle was at work in other aspects of life as well, though it was sometimes carried far beyond what was either necessary, called for, or appropriate. A few members of the gang had a strong tendency towards becoming quite violent, which made me as well as one or two others uneasy. It led to incidents where it could have been considered a plus in some ways, but it was escalating as we gotolder to the point where it was troublesome.

The most potentially violent member, and the unspoken leader, hardly looked the part at all. He was tall, thin, wore thick glasses, and had what could only be described as an innocent and angelic expression on his face. In addition he spoke in a deliberate, overly polite manner, particularly when he was on the edge of giving vent to an enormous rage. It could be scary, for he was also extremely strong and very adept in any kind of battle. There wasn't a better street fighter. Two incidents come to mind that capture how his leadership was carried out, and how valued it was in my early teenage years. By the same token it was what motivated me to leave the gang when I was seventeen by enlisting in the navy(this was during the second world war when many did the same, probably for patriotic reasons. There was no doubt that in my case it was a combination of not being able to imagine myself being drafted in the army, in conjunction with it being an easy way to leave the gang.)

The first incident concerned my exposure to an entirely different group and the effect it had in strengthening my attraction, while the intent was the opposite. A favored uncle was worried about the crowd I hung around with, both from their reputation(which I suspect was exaggerated) and from having seen them in the various athletic games he had watched. We had many conversations about it, as he tried everything he could think of to encourage me to join a jewish boys club he was associated with. Finally I agreed to give it a try. It seemed all right at first, because they were very interested in sports, which pleased me. Shortly after joining we travelled into a rough neighborhood to play a basketball game. We managed to just barely win, in spite of the obvious efforts to prevent it(the final thirty seconds must have been ten times longer). Upon leaving the gym it was immediately apparent that we were in for trouble as a hostile group approached us in a menacing way. Quick as a flash six of my teammates bolted into the car we had arrived in, locking the door, leaving one other and myself behind to deal with the assault. Fortunately the two of us survived by doing what we could, back to back, until police arrived upon the scene. I certainly understood how fear had taken over so that two of us were left, while the others were driven to protect themselves. It was just so counter to what I was accustomed to. Later at the next meeting of this group I tried to speak to it, insisting that we go back but this time prepared to stand together. They all thought I was foolish and would have none of it. It was crystal clear to me then why I was so drawn to my gang. There was simply no way they would have left for any reason. As an addendum, that was the end of my brief stay with that group and my gang gladly joined me in returning to play another game. The outcome of the game was the same, but not the aftermath. I'm sure an entirely different aura was silently communicated, for this group was, if anything, disappointed that there was no confrontation.

Another incident took place on our way to school, which was always an interesting experience. On the days the whole group drove, we all piled into an old
beatup clunker, and it was basically a miracle if we got there. All it took was for
one person to say let's not go today and that was it we were off on some kind of
adventure. This had happened so often that on this day we had resolved to end
up at school no matter what, and more than that to get there on time. One of the
streets we took was both busy and narrow. So there we were headed for school
pretty much on time when the car in front of us pulled in towards the curb to
pick someone up. The driver got out of the car leaving the back end sticking out
into the street so we couldn't pass .We all yelled and honked, but he acted like we
weren't there and refused to respond. The leader of our gang got out of the car
and in his most overly polite manner said, ""pardon me kind sir but I do believe
you have left your car blocking the street,and I am sure that you are pleased I am
calling it to your attention". Hearing that sound in his voice we all knew something was going to happen and that it could get unpleasant fast. The man unfortunately replied in a very abrupt and impatient fashion, "Hold your pants on kid.
It won't hurt you to wait until I'm ready". The leader appearing most angelic
stated, "I gather that is your final word on the matter...what a pity". He then
took over the wheel of the car, backed it up, and zoomed forward to crash right
into the side of what appeared to be a brand new car. Calmly he stepped out of
the car again, walked slowly up to the now stunned man whose jaw had dropped
open as if he couldn't believe what had happened. "Is there anything you would
like to say to me before I leave, I would be delighted to listen". I held my breath
and thankfully the man went to his car and moved it out of the way. It was this
kind of violence that was escalating as we got older, and though there was something positive in the refusal to be a victim, I thought there had to be better ways
toexpress it.

I really didn't fully appreciate how I was strengthening my own resolve never
to be a victim by being a part of such a gang. However, over the ensuing years I
was able to handle a host of difficult situations much more effectively as a consequence of that influence. Although I know there are times when Igo too far, I do
keep searching for those better ways. When I was in college, for example, I joined
a fraternity. I was a little surprised at my decision, because the demands for conformity and what I believed were false values permeated the atmosphere. However, it was the cheapest and most convenient source of room and board, and
when that was combined with their emphasis on a variety of sports it made the
decision easy. The first thing they did was assign me a mentor to teach me how to
dress. I actually thought it was funny, and didn't mind at all, because the person

was so genuine. Eventually he gave up on me as a hopeless case. There were other things that were very offensive to me, particularly the expectation that I would do something simply because it was either requested or ordered. That all ended one day when I was given the task of preparing the fraternity house for a party, since I was not going to attend it. The plan was to pick apples with a neighboring sorority and return to the house for cider and doughnuts in front of the fireplace. Noone asked, it was just assumed that because I was not going and hence given the assignment it would be done. This, in spite of the fact that I had made it clear on numerous occasions that I would in no way be responsive to such an approach.

The big day arrived, everyone left, and as I saw it I now had two options(the third of actually doing it was out of the question). The first was to simply ignore it and let the chips fall where they may. The second, which was very appealing (and reminiscent of my gang days), was to get my message across in an unmistakeable fashion. With the help of a friend we proceeded to totally lock and seal up the entire house from basement to attic, so that entry was impossible. This involved alot of work,(which was fun to do), including the boarding up and/or nailing shut of a large number of windows(locking and barricading the doors was easy). We had a ball enhanced when the whole group returned eager to warm up and enjoy the party only to find they couldn't gain entry. After realizing their shouts and threats were not being responded to, and their efforts to discover some weak spots were frustrated(we really did a good job), they began to appeal and bargain. By this time the girls had left to the chagrin of everyone. I then stated my purpose and as soon as they agreed to my conditions I opened the door.

The lessons I learned were also apparent in another arena, where I was the one a gang looked to as being the authority. This was of special interest to me because it gave me a chance to see things from a different perspective. While I was in medical school I applied for a job at a local boys club in order to make some money. The only opening they had was to teach tumbling to a gang of fourteen and fifteen year old boys. Even though I had no idea what it was, I implied that I could do it, and to my surprise I was hired instantly. I got a book from the library, read and practiced some moves, and went to the initial meeting where I discovered why I was hired so readily. This group of boys were in fact a gang and had been unmanageable. Several people had given up, believing they were incorrigible. So when I came along they decided to give it one more try.

The moment I greeted them I could see how they perceived me from their sullen, defiant looks. I also knew they would be testing me, though I didn't yet know exactly how. I was still under the impression that they had come to learn tumbling, so I began by repeating some things that I had so recently read about. One statement I made(from the book) was that once they learned how to fall properly they could drop from ten or fifteen feet without hurting themselves. That was all it took and the first test arrived. "Lets see you!". It was a moment of truth, which I would handle in a much different way today. At that time, however, with their eager and enthusiastic help, we put two tables and a chair one on top of the other and up I went. Holding my breath I dropped to the mat doing the best I could to follow the directions in the book. I landed with an awkward and jarring thud, obviously stunned, but not too badly hurt. Jumping to my feet I playfully exclaimed, "there nothing to it". They all cracked up laughing, as did I, and I then told them what I should have in the first place(and what I would now say instead of jumping). They could clearly see I didn't know anything about tumbling, but since I thought it was the only way I would get the job I let the staff think I did. I also thought if I did the best I could I might be able to teach them something. This led us into a discussion of what I did know to see if it matched with their interests. The result was in our forming a baseball team with me as the coach. It turned out to be a great experience for all of us. The boys club was also pleased, since it was the only time this particular gang had engaged in anything constructive.

A similar situation arose several years later when,as a fellow in child psychiatry, I volunteered to conduct group therapy in a local boys reform school. The room I was given was in the basement of an abandoned building, and the boys I was assigned to work with were waiting for me to arrive. Upon entering the room there was no mistaking the high level of tension. Before I could even sit down or introduce myself one of the boys approached me in a defiant and challenging manner. "You're in big trouble", he muttered. I pulled up a chair, sat down, and told him there was certainly no doubt about that. He continued in the same manner and I answered his questions grateful that we were talking. Gradually the other boys chimed in, especially when I would say something that surprised them. I was asked what I would do if they all attacked me; I simply replied that I had no idea . That answer intrigued all of them. I tried to explain that I certainly did not want to get hurt, nor did I want to hurt any of them, but I didn't know how I'd react until it happened. "Aren't you scared?", they wanted to know. Sure I told them, but I'd be much more scared if I didn't welcome what was happening right now. Silence fell over the room and from that moment the entire atmosphere changed. The sessions became a place to talk and try to understand. At one point they must have sensed something, for one boy asked me directly if I had ever been in a gang. My answer was a smile, as everyone knew his question was really a statement of feeling understood.

The world of medicine has changed enormously in recent years. Technological advances, as well as the deepening understanding of biophysiological processes, has grown beyond belief. Unfortunately the same cannot be said for a dedication to patient care, respect for autonomy, and search for what is right rather than cost effective. Those were qualities that once were taken for granted as the cornerstone that each physician aspired to attain. Of course there were always some who were blind to the healing power of such aspirations. The medical school class of 1948 was unique as a group, in that it was the first composed primarily of war veterans. Those members of the medical school faculty who remained tied to outdated ideas concerning the need for conformity had a great deal of difficulty with this class as a whole. There were frequent meetings in which what was seen as an insubordinate attitude was soundly criticized. Every moment of every day just seemed so terribly serious. Spontaneously a small group of individuals were drawn to each other, motivated by a search for some relief from the exaggerated sense of importance that was in the atmosphere everywhere. One could say that we formed a gang in which playing was the order of the day. I don't think a serious word was ever uttered between us. The best way to study for an exam, for example, was to play bridge and say a word in the subject at hand before making a bid. The supply of such words was quickly exhausted, and so others had to be found that taxed our creativity and left us roaring with laughter. Upon graduation we all went our separate ways.

Forty two years later, four members of that gang came together to play once again; and play we did. However, this time we all discovered that we had been attracted to each other not so much because of our playfulness, but more due to our idealistic dedication to being healers. Now we periodically had serious discussions, and stories to tell concerning our experiences during those forty two years. Some were humorous; some tragic ; some painful ; some joyous; yet overall they came from a deep devotion to finding and following what is right.

Gangs in general seem to bring out the best and worst in people. Terrorist gangs and many street gangs amply demonstrate how destructive they can be. Certainly the gang I joined in medical school nourished positive qualities in each of us, which made these qualities stronger as a result. The gangs from my developmental years were a combination of both. There appears to me to be a common theme in all the gangs I have come in contact with. This centers around the powerful impact of feeling the support and loyalty of others holding similar values. A problem arises either when there is something twisted in the shared value system, or when the hunger for belonging and feeling support overshadows every-thing else.

Beth

Having grown up in a world of deceit, self deception, outright lies, with only occasional truths(or more accurately half truths), not to mention the propensity to assign noble names to ignoble deeds, it is no wonder that I would be acutely sensitive to any situation in which these qualities were present. Fortunately I also had two major attachments that brought the shining light of integrity into my life(one a hassidic grandfather, the other an american indian woman; what an amazing combination). Retrospectively it explains so many of my reactions that, at the time they occurred, I had no idea of their meaning. The only thing that I noticed was feeling driven to expose shams wherever I saw them. Fortunately or unfortunately(sometimes it's hard to decide), there is a strong tendency to emphasize the point by in essence thumbing my nose at them .

I recall an incident when I was in the seventh grade that is illustrative. The school had an annual event called "backwards day". It was a special day in which the students took over the function of teachers, designed to demonstrate the difficulties of their task. Everyone looked forward to it as a fun-filled experience, as it usually meant watching a child struggle with trying to do an adequate job. There was no real time to prepare, since the assignments were not made until school began that day. Of course everyone held their breath, hoping to escape what had the potential of being quite embarrassing. Well I walked into the classroom to see my name written on the blackboard as the teacher for the day. My initial reaction was to feel stunned, but then the sham of pretending that I, in fact, had the authority of a teacher hit me. My answer then was simple and I enjoyed the moment immensely. "Class dismissed", was my declaration. Everyone left the premises laughing, leaving just me and the teacher staring at each other. I ended up in the principles office where I was bawled out, but it was worth it.

Another personal incident showed that same tendency even more clearly. I was riding in a huge limousine at the funeral of a grandfather I hardly knew, surrounded by grim faced, somber relatives, who from my perspective seemed to be trying very hard to appear sad. As far as I could tell all they succeeded in doing was to look dour and grumpy. I had often heard these same people speak of this grandfather in negative terms. My picture was of him constantly absorbed in listening to operas, oblivious to everything and everyone around him. Generally when I was with this group I spoke very little, so there I was at the age of twelve sitting quietly while we drove to the cemetery. Out of nowhere I suddenly began to sing a song fairly loud(I think I stunned everyone especially myself), "did you ever think when the hearse went by...that you would be the next to die...the worms crawl in...the worms crawl out...the worms play pinochle on your snout......". The looks that then came my way made me want to disappear; but as I look back it pleases me that I had expressed myself so vividly.

In addition I have been told I had a firm, determined sense of what belonged to me from the time I was quite young. This was reflected in a story that may or may not have been true(I can never be sure as to which when being told stories). Whether it is, or isn't, it does capture a feeling I can recall from as far back as I can remember. Apparently at the age of one year I was handed a penny to give to an organ grinder's monkey. When the monkey took it, I set out in a relentless pursuit until I got it back. I do believe also that I intuitively knew it wasn't only material objects(like the penny) that could be taken. Much more important were the validity and credibility of one's perceptions. Young children can be particularly vulnerable to this form of robbery, though not so much when it is blatant and unmistakeable. However, they may then be forced to either hide or disguise these perceptions(usually of deceit or betrayal)so it can only emerge in indirect ways. The various experiences that exposed me to the destructive influence of deception also made me much more aware of these subtle expressions of the perception of deceit.What I apparently had found necessary to put into action is thus most frequently expressed in quieter ways. Although some may be communicated directly and explicitly, the most significant are usually expressed through dreams, fantasies, indirect references contained in narrative stories, and what is often referred to as magical thinking.

I have wondered why it was that dreams, fantasies, made-up stories, and magical thinking are so often treated as if they had no relationship to anything that could be thought of as real. It's really quite surprising, since fairy tales, for example, are known to convey some powerful truths about the human condition. Furthermore we have no trouble recognizing the true picture a caricature can portray. Yet when it comes to considering what truths these mental productions contain, there is a strong tendency to relegate them to imagination(which they are)as if this was a reason to deny any connection to what is actually true. Even as a child I thought it was puzzling when someone would say "oh, that's all in your head". The implication was that the particular experience could be somewhere else(I somehow knew even a sore foot was in my head). More to the point I did know they meant if you couldn't see it, or touch it, you must have imagined it. The part I couldn't see(and still can't)was why that by definition signified that there was nothing either valid or real involved.

At the time I was in psychoanalytic training, there was what I considered to be a strange understanding of the role of fantasy in a person's life and in treatment. There was no doubt of its power and great significance, but it was exclusively seen in the light of the distortions that it created. Thus fantasies and dreams were sought out and explored in depth, though practically never for the truths they revealed. What seemed obvious to me was actively denied, as if the idea of a fantasy or dream reflecting what was actual, real, or truthful was in itself a fantasy. This in the face of a particular phenomena that was disturbing to me in the way it was ignored. I seriously questioned imposing the conditions of psychoanalytic treatment in place of discovering them. Yet in case after case the same theme was repeated of having to submit to the demands of much needed others, with no seeming awareness of its applicability to the treatment. Along with this theme, whenever other associations appeared that readily fit into treasured theoretical concepts they were attended to as the only ones of any importance. It soon became clear to me (and others as well)that this way of perceiving a patients productions actually prevented(and thereby protected)the analyst from seeing the part he or she played in what was happening between them. How ironic that the person advocating a devotion to the truth turns out then to be violating that very principle in the way the relationship is understood and managed(fortunately today this serious self deception has been recognized and in some quarters corrected).

My first experience in conducting a "proper psychoanalytic" treatment(interestingly labelled a "control" case), acquainted me with how readily I could slide into becoming brainwashed(more accurately brain poisoned). My patient was using the couch for the first time after a series of evaluative interviews. He was extremely anxious as he was faced with lying down out of my sight, which I knew from our earlier contact was especially difficult for him(a phobic reaction to a supine position was one of his symptoms). Yet when he began asking a flurry of questions, to my astonishment I could hardly believe the words that came out of my mouth. "What makes you ask", is what I said. The absurdity of my response struck me, and I couldn't contain my laughter. When I explained how funny I sounded to myself, we both could be more relaxed in exploring the source of his anxiety.

During this period of time the world of fantasy and dreams was opening up to me, expanding my vision of their messages in a whole host of directions. Much of what I had learned did not appear to be entirely accurate, as I gained a deeper appreciation of the stories they contained. I had been taught that a major function of a dream was to disguise hidden wishes, as well as hidden truths. My impression was that there may be times when the motive is to disguise, but much more frequently their purpose is to reveal those truths. However, they were doing so in a different language; the language of symbols. If that language is not understood, the motive could easily be misperceived. It also became noticeable to me that, especially with children, it was often the only language available to communicate the existence of lies, deception, injustices, and other negative qualities associated with much needed adults. This was quite a revelation, because it was applicable to the position I occupied with my patients(children of all ages) and I had to notice how often I unknowingly introduced these kinds of negative experiences. I felt like I had been presented with a key, which liberated me from perpetuating areas of darkness. Seeing things in this new light changed my entire attitude. Instead of searching for how a patient was in essence wrong, I found myself listening for how they were right. Consequently, my task was not to show someone how they had distorted an experience in order to demonstrate that they were wrong; rather it was to discover with them how they had seen something usually without realizing it. From that position both of us could then easily see where the distortions were present and how they came about. A therapeutic relationship is not meant to be adversarial, and when it is something is wrong.

I began to examine more closely various concepts that I had taken for granted, yet sensed there was more than what appeared on the surface. From my background and what I was learning my attention was drawn to magical thinking. Whenever it emerged within a patient it was generally explained away as a product of immaturity, probably reflecting the response to a regression. This was certainly true as a description, but not enough of an explanation. The deeper significance that this type of thinking possesses is hinted at in the root meaning of the word magic: the art of employing natural powers to produce effects apparently supernatural. Fortunately my eyes were open when Beth, as if by magic, came onto the scene to show me the power and vital communication contained in magical thinking.

She was a remarkably bright and articulate three year old child, which made the lessons she had to teach extremely clear. Even the way she was referred was unusual, in that she had asked her parents to find her a doctor who could help with her trouble. She had been complaining for several months of severe stomach aches and occasional episodes of vomiting with no apparent physical reason. Her parents were quite psychologically minded and thought she was upset about her mother's pregnancy, anticipating that she would be displaced. When they first told her of the pregnancy she had seemed pleased, and began to pretend that she too, like her mother, was pregnant. Initially they had seen it as cute, but as time went on and she showed signs of believing she actually did have a baby inside of her, they started to worry. She got increasingly upset, they were at a loss as to how to comfort or reassure her, and she then wanted them to take her to a doctor.

In she walked without a moments hesitation, looking very poised and proud of herself. Then, in a serious and emphatic manner, she informed me that she just knew she had a baby in her tummy. Furthermore the only way it could come out was through her mouth. She had thought and thought about it, but just couldn't figure out how to do it. That's why she came to see me—to find a way to help her get it out. She had tried to force it out, but only threw up. It made her tummy feel even worse. Pausing, she asked if I believed there was a baby inside of her. Her question really caught my attention, because it not only implied that I might not believe her, but also that she was accustomed to meeting disbelief in others. To pretend I did, if I did not, would be condescending, and as such be hurtful. What a wonderful vehicle for probing as to whether I would be straight with her, and in what category I belonged. I could honestly say, in the context of what I had come to know, that I was curious as to how she was right. Therefore I asked her why it was a question, since so far she hadn't given me any indication that I shouldn't believe her.

She explained that everyone she met thought she made it all up. Her parents tried to tell her how babies are made and born, and how it was impossible for a baby to really be there. They didn't believe it and worse didn't know how to get it out. Tears welled up in her eyes as she described what hurt so much. The baby wasn't a part of her; that's what made it so scary. It could grow bigger and even eat her up. While I listened, I thought the baby really was already doing all of that. The feelings associated with her fantasy were not yet integrated and thus experienced as a foreign body. They also occupied so much of her energy and attention as time went on that they were growing bigger. What was true in her magical thinking as to how the baby was to be delivered was as yet unknown. She looked up at me and in an anguished voice asked if I had any idea of how to do it.

I told her that since she was convinced it had to come out of her mouth, we had an important clue, so we would have to figure out what that meant. She immediately caught on and was intrigued. She then started to list everything she could think of that came out of her mouth; food, spitting, vomiting.....and suddenly her eyes lit up......Words!!. We both laughed and I remarked that she really found something that felt right. She thought so too, got very excited, but then stopped short with a puzzled look on her face. I said that she had shown me how much she wanted to do things herself, but now that we had found where to search we still didn't know exactly what would do it. It appeared to me like she would need my help, for it wasn't just any words. We had to find the ones that fit, so they could bring the baby out. She nodded yes vigorously,appearing relieved. We agreed to keep meeting until we found them.

Simply by being able to talk freely, knowing that I truly believed in the reality of fantasies and magical thinking, she had come upon the striking idea that words were the means by which the baby could be delivered. She felt the push of feelings seeking to be expressed, only having her fantasies and magical thinking as a means of doing so. One involved the baby, and the other the proper words to deliver it. To cast them aside as unreal could only result from a narrow view of reality, something this child knew quite well even in the face of others disbelief. The right words were not yet known, and my task was to provide the opportunity for them to emerge. She was eager to talk and the first thing that occurred to her was her wish to clear up the confusion in her mind as to how babies were made. She couldn't quite grasp what it meant that her daddy put a seed into her mommy where it met an egg and grew into a baby in a special place. This made her think that she had swallowed one of his seeds. With that she paused, took a deep breath, and almost shouted out; "I don't want the baby!". The force with which these words were spoken caught her by surprise. It was quite a moment; for I thought the process of delivering the baby had just begun.

I commented on the angry sound in her voice and she launched into a tirade about all of the changes in her life. Her mother was always too tired to play with her, everyone was excited about the pregnancy, and she hated it. This went on for several weeks. At times she was so furious that her face got red as though she could barely contain it. There were other times when she expressed it playfully, enjoying the idea of making her parents be as hurt as she was. Through all of this, there was no mention of the baby inside of her. At this point we missed a session due to the new baby's arrival.

She returned looking subdued and in a barely audible voice mumbled that she supposed I wanted to hear about her baby sister, before bursting forth with incidents centering around her reactions to the baby. I alluded to her wishing she could be a baby, which made her stop for a second to nod her head yes before changing it to an emphatic no. She then smiled broadly stating how good it felt to be bigger. Almost as an afterthought she casually mentioned that the baby inside of her was gone. With a pensive expression she began to tell me what was so awful for her before the baby was born. Everytime she saw her mother's tummy getting bigger it gave her a sick feeling inside. The whole idea of her parents doing something together that excluded her, with this being the result, was more than she could stand. Whenever it came into her mind the only way she could ease the pain was to imagine her daddy making a baby with her.

So there it was. She delivered the baby and her secret was out. Once she was able to give vent to her hostility, though it was not openly evident as it was taking place, the baby inside of her was being delivered along with her angry words. Her casual reference to the momentous event of the disappearance of her symptom was interesting. On closer inspection this attitude on her part made alot of sense, for in giving up the symptom what it was designed to defend her against rose to the surface. She not only had to swallow her aggressive feelings(the seed), but she also was holding the more threatening fantasies out of her awareness(the growing baby). Her greatest anxiety was connected to her fantasy of her parents engaged in hidden activities(having sexual overtones), from which she was excluded. The implied betrayal, as well as the overstimulation and curiosity, added to the threat. Although her initial anxiety was temporarily relieved by imagining her father making a baby with her, it became a source of even greater trouble. Now that it was accessible to her, the accompanying feelings could be absorbed and integrated.

Some important principles were clearly highlighted in the experience with Beth. Arguments as to whether a given event was real or imagined fade into the background, as the question of what story each has to tell moves into prominence. A photograph can only show so much, whereas a caricature can bring out what is otherwise hidden: to get the full picture both are necessary. Dreams, fantasies, and magical thinking all carry symbolic messages having the potential to expose hidden truths. They do so because they serve so well as an antidote to the impact of destructive interactions. Therefore they play a vital role in gaining a deeper appreciation of what is real.

Hope

Prior to September 11th. I thought about states of mind like hope and despair either in relation to patients, or on those occasions when it was relevant with family and friends. On that fateful day, the world was changed forever. One effect that I noticed was in a desire to shed light upon how I could remain hopeful in the face of such a horrible incident. My attention was then focused on describing the experiences that had been instrumental in shaping my understanding of what kinds of forces seemed to keep hope alive.

Who knows where something actually begins. When I was about 9 or 10 years old,however, I can recall puzzling over the question of why I should be afraid of dying. It was clearly a part of life, so why did it seem so frightening? In my imagination the fear centered around the sensation of no longer seeing or knowing anything or anyone in the world as I did at that moment. It was as though my entire experience of myself had suddenly and irrevocably been removed. Over time I was able to both welcome and stay with the fearful sensation long enough to become more discriminating, and it seemed to me that it was exactly how I felt whenever a situation arose where my fear and anxiety carried me away from, and out of touch with, my usual way of reacting and responding. It was not a big jump to then notice that the fear of dying, for me at least, was based upon the experience of losing my hold on the particular qualities that characterized me as a human being.

Early in my career, I was especially blessed in establishing contact with a small number of unique children. They were amazingly adept at teaching me how to identify truth and lies in human relationships, and in particular even the slightest of self deceptions on my part. Although each was quite different, they could be classified as (what was known at the time) primary infantile autism(in contrast to autistic behavior secondary to brain damage or so called Asberger's syndrome). In the presence of any form of deceptiveness, their reactions were quite extreme; from total and complete withdrawal to other behavior making it unmistakeable that something was terribly wrong. There was never a doubt when any sort of lie was in the air. In addition,during the course of their treatment, they exhibited a similar pattern of growth suggesting that I was observing and participating in something universal in human development having to do specifically with the preverbal years.

Initially they did not display any evidence of what could be thought of as anxiety or panic, until they relinquished their autistic posture. At that point they felt enormously vulnerable, as panic dominated the scene. My participation was then essential in being able to bring true hope with absolutely no trace of anything they could interpret as false reassurance. It was easy for me to falter, as I often did, in negotiating such terrain. Timing was vital, for at some moments it meant being able to physically buffer their terrorized experience while at other moments it required my standing firm in offering them the opportunity to absorb as fully as possible what was happening. These were the important steps they were taking towards learning to integrate the meaning of the severe trauma they were reexperiencing.

Fortunately with each I had an earlier event occurring between us that gave me a degree of guidance, which involved another characteristic of the initial sessions. Surprisingly a dramatic happening appeared, seemingly out of the blue, having enormous implications for what was to follow. In one, for example, after two sessions of pacing and gesturing with his fingers, giving no indication of being receptive to any of my efforts to reach him, he suddenly turned to me and stated "are you listening?". This from a child who had never shown any capacity towards language development, but also appearing at the precise instant when my mind had wandered and in fact I was not listening. Another spent two sessions doing nothing other than crawling on the floor gathering lint, grunting as he did so. At the end of the third session, as I was trying to help him get up to leave, he muttered "if you want to help me you're going to have to kill my mother". A third was a child who had been almost totally immobilized everywhere, to the point that he would sit in one place all day unless he was moved. From the second he crossed the doorsill to enter my office he became a bundle of energy, throwing himself from one position to another, jabbering away non-stop using unintelligible sounds. I finally grasped one word, which I then repeated, and he became so excited it looked like he had just received the greatest gift in the world. Later he just casually remarked that he had never found anyone he wanted to talk to, or be with,before.

With each of these children, sometimes I had to hold them gently, close the windows to soften the noise from outside, or turn out the lights. Everything was much too painful to bear. At other times I had to speak about my understanding of what they were going through and not in anyway interfere with, or attempt to soften, the blows. They indicated, mostly by their actions, how much it meant to them for me to recognize all the real dangers they were confronted with in the outer world. Only then could I speak to the greater dangers that they faced in their internal world. Although they were able to grow considerably in some limited areas, they had to be able to incorporate the panic (in essence have the experience of allowing it to emerge and permeate their being and then actually find they were bigger so it could be contained) before they could then move into the biggest step of all. This was to possess as their own the confident knowledge that the pathway of reaching wholeness as a separate person was completely in their hands. This achievement was everything—all else paled in comparison. Genuine hope was now theirs.

This is the tragedy of pre-verbal traumas. They are endlessly present in the foundation of the personality with no access to being represented. The impact then has no access to gaining integration into the total fabric of the prsonality. There simply is no doorway to having exposure to more advanced functions. Hence the awful dilemma of needing somehow to find a way to make these traumas representable, so they can be integrated, yet not be repeated and increase the accompanying despair. Is psychotherapy the only way, or even a viable way, to approach such a matter? The mind and body are a single entity so how can a relationship be the vehicle? In my opinion there can be no interpersonal techniques(they are artificial and thus untrustable), or even so-called perfect intuneness, if indeed such can exist(two separate individuals would of necessity have moments of a lack of fit, not to mention the inevitable blind spots). So how could a relationship provide the necessary experience of a repetition of the trauma, while at the same time offering a different outcome? To enter a pychotherapeutic relationship with the intent of creating such a repetition would be far too destructive to even allow any integration. The struggle goes on searching for a solution, and I do not know the answer. I can only go by my experience, which tells me it is well worth the effort. A key element is my own unwavering devotion to finding the truth; first and foremost of what my contribution has been, but also to see what my patient brings. They both go together. Anything that transpires comes to no good end without both elements being in the picture.

All of this is a preamble to the larger question of what I consider to be hope in the context of the world we live in. As far as I can see the external world has the potential for every conceivable aspect of life . There are opportunities for love, integrity, courage, constructive growth, teamwork, and every other positive quality one can think of. At the same time there are also opportunities for hatred, indifference, cowardice, deceptions, destructive acts of all kinds, ugly collusions, and every other negative quality imagineable. Any conceivable possibility is available for people to be lured into, choose to be imposed upon,or selected,and it is not always clear which is which. To me it is particularly unnerving when I come in contact with what appear to be ignoble deeds being given noble names. Sometimes it is patently evident, but at other times there are grey areas and not enough may be known to make the distinction. Welcoming such a challenge, of trying to find and bring clarity in the face of ambiguity and uncertainty, I believe to be a necessary ingredient if hope is to have a foundation to grow upon. However, it can be like fighting windmills if there isn't an associated search within for any influences at work to distort what is perceived. We cannot help but be influenced by our experiences in life, though there is a significant difference between having them be a source of information rather than a force that obscures and/or skews our vision. In this regard it seems to me if there is to be hope in this world, it grows out of,and depends upon, our doing whatever we can to be as whole, honest and forthright as it is possible to be. We must also recognize that there may very well be limits to how successful we can be. It is under these kinds of conditions that attitude means everything; not as a fixed, forced, or will power determined stance, but as a deep awareness of the power evolving out of gaining access to the most buried, hidden, and darkest parts of our being. Whether we achieve success in this journey at any given moment is not the issue. The power rests in opening ourselves to genuinely being receptive to the opportunity of owning what is ours, including what may be considered as evil or destructive. We will then have reached the terrorist in his or her hiding place, not with the desire to destroy but to transform, and thus increase the positive energy available to us(as well as whatever contribution it makes to the forces in the surrounding atmosphere).

When my children came to me in distress over some disturbing episode in their lives, my tendency was to try to comfort them by offering what I considered to be true reassurance at the time. Depending on the circumstances it might have taken the form of advice, providing a missing perspective, or simply listening. Now I see these incidents somewhat differently, and I think I missed many golden opportunities to give something much more important. When my grandchildren are distressed over some injustice, rejection, hurt feelings, failure, or any other outside occurence, my immediate reaction, as well as my perspective, has changed. The first thing that jumps into my mind is what a wonderful opportunity they have been presented with to learn more about themselves. I introduce it by saying that outside matters can certainly get worse, and usually do, followed by an explanation of what I consider to be most valuable to them. In welcoming whatever comes their way, especially how it affects them and how they may have either created or participated in whatever happened, a potential doorway is opened to retrieve things they have relegated to the darkness. This would be particularly vital in regard to feelings that are painful to see or frightening to encounter. They might, or might not, gain insight into their meaning, but the fact that they have searched makes a lasting impact. It is at the very least a step in the right direction. In their moving in this fashion, the possibility of genuine hope begins to emerge and with it an opening for becoming all that is in them to be(a lifetime journey at best). The consequences of such an approach, in my opinion, reach out far beyond what is visible and offers a measure of hope for the world at large as well.

The impact of September 11th. resonates within me in a variety of directions. First and foremost is the incident itself. The complete lack of humane feelings, the nature and horrifying vision of innocent victims blasted to pieces or confronted with a Hobson's choice of ways to end their lives, the overwhelming sadness of the losses, and the absolute devastation possible for a few insane fanatics to create on such a large scale is simply hard to take in . Then there is the aftermath of realizing its implications. Even Pollyanna would have trouble finding a positive meaning to this one;although there have been some positive consequences. The best that I can see is of it representing a wakeup call: to look closely at how we conduct ourselves. In what subtle ways are we terrorists to ourselves or others, and how can we transform what we discover into constructive, growth promoting pursuits? An imposing task to be sure, for the answers may come slowly or perhaps not at all. The point is that the search itself can be rewarding, but if it is not recognized as a meaningful option a significant opportunity is lost.

Because of my background I was also drawn to noticing the similarities between the terrorists declarations and the ceremony of Passover. An escalating series of plagues were visited on the Egyptians, in the name of God, demanding that the Jewish people be released from slavery. When these warnings were ignored a final drastic step was taken to kill Egyptian firstborn infants before that freedom was granted. Of course there are some important differences, but nevertheless it does speak to the need to root out such destructive forces whereever they exist, not just in the "enemy's" backyard. Although the name of God may be invoked, the name is emanating from man. The essence of what is derived from whatever God represents is expressed in the principles that guide our lives. When these principles deviate from what we know are positive qualities(love, truth, integrity, genuine care giving, courage, creativity, beauty etc) they must be examined so that the twists and distortions can be straightened out.

I also could not help but recall the story of Abraham's relationship to what he thought of as God. His readiness to demonstrate his faith in God by killing his son Isaac, from my perspective can only be viewed as his failing the test. The most interesting facet in light of the current tragedy seems to me to involve Abraham's influence on his two sons. One, Ishmael, fathered the line of Arabs, while Isaac carried the knowledge of his fathers willingness to kill him as an unhealed wound passed on to his Jewish descendents. Both sons knew of their fathers destructiveness and carried it in two different directions.

What was brought to our attention so dramatically and unmistakeably on September 11th. has always been present in the world. Sadly, but maybe fortunately, it required exposing a supposedly powerful, strong, free, humane society to the terrible consequences of ignoring destructiveness for the problem to be seriously addressed. It is now crystal clear to everyone that an answer must be found, and the resources are potentially available to support it. We can no longer afford to close our eyes to terrorism wherever it is; in the macrocosm of the world or the microcosm of our individual being. The recognition itself is a good beginning, which brings with it genuine hope. The pathway must continue to be travelled, probably forever, undoubtedly with many obstacles along the way. It is simply the right thing to do, and the rewards are enormous.

The usual definition of hope refers to the expectation of something good or desireable to happen; whereas the root meaning makes reference to having a feeling of trust, the ability to rely, and to be confident. Although we may have some influence on outside events, there is no way we can control them as September11th. so amply demonstrates. However, the potential for establishing integration, trust, the ability to rely(especially upon ourselves), and to have a solid sense of confidence is always there to work towards internally. Once we are on such a path, and truly know it, there, of course, would be the expectation of something good and desirable to happen.

Good Enough

At first glance the words good enough seem like a strange way to describe a most desired goal in human relationships. Upon taking a second look(the root meaning of respect), a clearer picture emerges. Whenever two separate and unique human beings engage in a relationship it is inevitable for there to be moments when they are simply out of touch with each other. It cannot be otherwise, unless one became an extension of the other, in which case they would no longer be separate(and each would lose their uniqueness in the process). In addition probably noone, in our complex society, emerges unscathed from the demands of development, so that blind spots remain. Any meaningful attachments, by their very nature, would undoubtedly activate childhood injuries in one way or another interfering with clarity and perspective. The fact that these moments of a lack of fit occur is not, in and of itself, a problem. Provided the relationship has contained a sufficient degree of intuneness to be trustable, these troublesome experiences offer a wonderful opportunity for each party to learn. In fact there is no greater stimulus to the emergence of latent resources and hence to facilitate growth. This is precisely why good enough is the very best we can offer to someone we care about.

I have been asked a number of times over the years as to who my role models were. For some reason I found it a hard question to answer. I knew some people who had been very helpful to me, and others I admired greatly, but the words just did not fit. It took a long time before I could see why. Intuitively I had a deep appreciation for the value of "good enough", and as soon as I realized it, the knowledge of who my role model was moved right up to the forefront of my mind. It makes me smile when I think about it, since in saying it out loud(or writing it) it sounds or looks like I'm joking. However, I know how true it is, and I'm sure people who know me would nod their head in agreement. That wonderful cartoon character, Mr. Magoo, bumping into walls because he cannot see, is exactly what I feel like in those situations where I am blind. I also believe I am open to learning, can ultimately notice when I am bumping into walls, and value finding the truth. Consequently I consider myself to be good enough, and look to Mr. Magoo to remind me of my task.

Early in my training, before I had any idea of how much there was to learn, I had no usable concept of what good enough meant. Nevertheless as I look back I can see that I was slowly discovering it. I recall meeting with an overly polite older man, who kept apologizing for everything he did that seemed in the least bit out of place. He was sorry for perhaps choosing the wrong chair when he sat down, for accidently brushing his arm against my desk, for having dragged in a piece of dirt on his shoe, and for almost anything else that caught his attention. His primary complaint, which he repeated endlessly, was that no matter where he went or what he did noone seemed to like him. He droned on and on with a flat, monotonous tone in his voice. I listened trying to find something I could say that might be helpful, but I found myself feeling somewhat annoyed and irritated. I did not appreciate at the time how important it was to pay attention to such feelings, believing they were intrusive and had to be pushed aside or ignored. In my attempt to be therapeutic, I was formulating a question to ask him as to whether he had considered the part he might play in the way others reacted. What popped out of my mouth, both to his and my astonishment, was; "how can anyone like you?". We stared at each other for a moment and I didn't quite know what to say, so I just shrugged my shoulders. He looked down mumbling, "you too eh?". I could only say yes and then try as best as I could to describe why. To my utter amazement he opened up and showed a part of himself I had no idea existed. There in front of me was a frightened little boy, talking to a cruel, demeaning, perfection demanding mother. In the background was his deep pain at the loss of a much loved, but passive and intimidated father, who had died in an automobile accident. At any rate without knowing it I had been good enough; the lack of fit became apparent to both of us as my irritation burst forth. Associated with it a door was opened for a genuine interaction. I showed my willingness to acknowledge the truth of my feeling about him, and he accepted this as an invitation for him to also speak the truth. What then came forward was the deeper feelings he harbored toward some painful experiences from early in his life.

Children can be such good teachers, particularly if they have a receptive audience. Of course there may be moments where there is little awareness that a message is being communicated. In that case whatever avenue they have chosen may have to escalate until it gets across. Sadly, if it is not received the potential for learning and growth is lost. In this regard, I'm reminded of a penetrating lesson taught to me by a then two and a half year old daughter. I had just returned home from visiting my wife and newborn infant in the hospital. Flushed with excitement over the addition to our family, there was nothing else on my mind as I greeted her. She, however, was extremely upset and in no mood to listen to me tell her about the experience. Everything she touched was frustrating, as she peri-odically erupted into explosive temper tantrums. I knew she was reacting to the changes in her life and all of the feelings it aroused, so I directed all of my energy into encouraging her to talk about it. The more I talked, the more irritable she became, and the more I thought it was essential to reach some mutual under-standing of what was happening. What an awful vicious cycle ; there I was like Mr. Magoo blindly bumping into walls. It didn't dawn on me how out of tune I was. Fortunately she was persistent, and as the intensity of her frustration esca-lated I slowly began to realize how far off the mark I was.

My child not only refused to accept any of my "thoughtful" and "insightful" words, but also was determined to discourage this kind of communication. The incident took place when I was in the midst of my psychiatric training, all wrapped up in the occupational hazzard of believing that the psychological con-cepts I was learning were useful and applicable in all circumstances. I hadn't yet noticed how talking and understanding could be used to create emotional dis-tance. Yet that was exactly what I was doing, and my daughter in her unique way was doing everything possible to get through to me. Although I was calm and outwardly unmoved by her outbursts, inwardly I was registering the futility of my words and searching for something that would bridge the gap(I was learning). At that point she must have sensed the change in my attitude, for she looked me straight in the eye with a penetrating gaze and said, "why don't you spank me already!"

Her words made a huge impact, as my eyes opened to see a picture thatI had avoided. She was obviously feeling overwhelmed by the events taking place with the birth of another child(the third in less than three years). Underneath my excitement, the pain she was experiencing was resonating with my own. Inadvert-ently, I was pushing it away in order to bring her my idea of the understanding she was lacking. No doubt I was secretly hoping she would do the same. Instead she was teaching me that the moment could only be shared by making the trou-blesome feelings I also was struggling with known to her. An incredible lesson to be sure, but I didn't have all the words myself as yet. What was now clear was her need to break through the barrier that I had created with my big words. My insis-tence upon talking only heightened her frustration, finally resulting in her demand for me to spank her. She certainly was pointing out a direction, since she had been driven to cry out for the only thing she could think of that might meet her urgent need for emotional contact. At last I had the opportunity to answer her request, though I was not capable of honoring it in the form she presented. I held her closely, as our feelings were exchanged wordlessly. She looked satisfied because she had established the contact she was searching for, and in addition had been effective in getting her message across. I was pleased in regard to what I had discovered about myself, and in learning what it meant to be good enough.

Although the nature of a relationship determines what conditions are necessary to foster growth, the principles guiding those conditions are the same. It may not always be possible to recognize what is, or isn't, good enough. Often the fear of losing a needed figure may be so imposing that the necessary actions cannot be permitted, while the person looked to for guidance may not be able to see, The adversarial qualities of the resulting interaction is in itself a clue. However, even then there may not be any clear direction to follow. It is here that the language of symbols can be a big help, and nothing is more expressive than what appears in a dream. Early in my career I was gradually becoming aware of just how much a patient perceived about the significance of my behavior, without fully realizing it. The enormous effect of the manner in which I introduced the conditions of the treatment was particularly noticeable. With this in mind I listened closely to see if this was also true with others beside myself. In case after case it stood out most strikingly in regard to what was called the fundamental principle of "free association". Interesting, the idea was to emphasize the importance of having the freedom to say whatever came to mind. Yet it was applied either as an actual instruction, which implicitly or even explicitly demanded conformity; or as a suggestion, which had a seductive quality and was often received with distrust.

What I observed so frequently was a patients perception of the actual behavior of an analyst treated as though it was a fantasy distortion. Afterwards the entire thrust of the relationship was occupied with conflicts around autonomy, submission to authority, and seductiveness. Thus it seemed evident to me that this basic principle, the cornerstone upon which the special qualities of psychoanalytic treatment were based, should be introduced through the avenue of how an analyst participated. Then an alliance could truly be built on a bond of mutual purpose in searching for the truth. On the patient's side this would consist of providing, through free associations, the unrecognized knowledge of what was needed to grow. On the analyst's side was the interpretation of that message, and use of it in managing the treatment. I no longer presented a direction to report all psychic content without using censorship or judgement. First because it placed the foundation of the treatment on an illusory basis, since it was impossible to follow. In addition it depended upon submission or conformity for its success. These were the very attitudes it was vital to eliminate in order to create the proper conditions for growth to unfold. I adopted a listening posture and introduced the principle of free association by simply interpreting whatever I heard that had relevance to this mode of communication.

In the midst of this change in my approach, a young man sought help with what he initially described as a mild case of impotence. It later turned out that he had been suffering from total ejaculatory impotence, but the humiliation he felt was so extreme he could barely admit it to himself. The early sessions were filled with his frantic pleas for direction and guidance. All he wanted from me was to tell him exactly what to do, when, and how. He kept complaining about a lack of purpose, angrily insisting that left to his own devices he would travel in never ending circles. Once he got caught up in them he was only led into an overwhelming state of frustration and despair. This, in fact, seemed to be an apt portrayal of what was happening. However, I understood(and interpreted)his demands as an expression of his enormous fear of following his spontaneous thoughts and feelings, and of revealing some as yet unspoken fantasies about our relationship. When this patient protested loudly against that idea, combined with his experience of the relationship as offering him no guidance, it raised many doubts, questions and uncertainty as to the accuracy of my understanding(not to mention the efficacy of how I was participating). I even began to think that I had made a mistake. Perhaps this was a situation that called for the standard, classical psychoanalytic position of giving explicit directions. At this juncture he reported the following dream:

"I was travelling on a road, lost and confused, desperately needing to get to Williamsburg. At first the road was deserted, but I noticed a raggety-looking hobo standing at the side of the road. He appeared to be familiar with the surroundings, so I asked him for directions to my destination. He merely replied that I should follow the road. I saw many roads and asked which one. With quiet conviction he told me to take any road, they would all get me there.. I was surprised that my fear lessened, and I knew that he was right".

The dream reflected his perception of my attitude, and of it pointing the way to reach what he so desparately needed. This despite his conscious experience being almost the opposite. The image of the hobo was an interesting portrayal of how he saw me. In part it revealed his efforts to depreciate my contribution, and in part to a secret he later brought out that validated my sensing he was harboring an unspoken fantasy about me(he had been driving by my house and observing me with my children, usually dressed much like the hobo). In addition the city he was searching for carried his own name, as if to underscore what he truly had to find. At any rate the dream communicated what he could not, and it assured me that I was being good enough.

The rewards that I have reaped from appreciating the value of being good enough have been enormous in every aspect of my life. In my work it heightened my awareness of the significance of my contribution to the relationship with my patients, especially in those moments when I was feeling like Mr. Magoo. Elements that I intuitively sensed as being essential became more solidly present within me, much to the benefit of those I worked with as well as myself. Because I could see with clarity how hurtful it was to sacrifice one's self in a relationship, I was open to, and welcomed, receiving phone calls at any time. It simply was not a problem, for if I was not receptive I saw the value of communicating my reaction. An opening was now available for both of us to learn, an opportunity that would be unfair of me to expect my patient to even notice much less take responsibility for. If the call was driven from something destructive in the patient, it was now in a place where it could be addressed. If the call was touching something in me that had been hidden, it was now accessible. Finally if it was a constructive motive seeking to further growth, could there be a better way than to receive it?. Perhaps most important of all, it was clear to me that if patients were going to feel safe enough to open up areas of vulnerability they were entitled to know how they were being received. Revealing potential blind spots is a significant part of being good enough.

A teenage granddaughter was given an assignment in school to write a character sketch of someone in her life. She chose me as that person. The essay she produced was sent to me and I was so deeply touched by her words that I immediately sat down and wrote her one in response. These two essays placed together, to me vividly give expression to the essence of what good enough means.

PAWPAW

A doctor, a friend, a person hated by some and loved by others, but to my siblings and I he is a grandpa. We call him PawPaw, although he never forced this, he has always wanted us to call him anything we choose. These names ranged from Doc, to Grandpa, to even his real name, Roy. When I was just a little girl, I was the closest to him. His perspective on life was ideal to me. Although we've grown apart over the years, he is still a role model of mine and I have many reasons for simply loving him.

He stands at approximately five feet, five inches tall. The little hair he has left makes a ring around his head. At nearly seventy five years old, he has the muscle of a twenty year old and the heart of a child. My intuition tells me this is how it shall remain forever. Four days a week when he goes to work, he dresses in the same suits he wore in 1970. These consist of either black or gray pants and jacket with a clip-on tie. Fashionable? In his own way I suppose.

From the beginning I was close to PawPaw. For a reason not of importance I held resentment against my own father, so PawPaw was the closest man to me. There is a special bond we share, because of this, now. I always cried when I was a baby, and the only people able to hush my tears were my mom and PawPaw. My mother simply had to rock me, but PawPaw was successful by singing me dirty limericks.

"There once was a man from Nantucket...." he sang.

As I got older this ended, but other traditions began. I'm sure, though, if I asked, he would gladly hold me and sing to me again.

Up to this day, whenever we see each other we become the "breakfast club-bers". That is, we wake up early and he takes whoever is awake, out to eat. Every Christmas, I wake up looking forward to the giant stocking filled with presents of t-shirts, candy, and calendars. Lately, as I grow older, my mom realizes that I don't need this anymore, so we don't fly back to St. Louis, where he lives, for the holidays. Moving away makes you miss things like this. No longer do we go to brunch every Sunday or have family dinners every Friday night, I have survived, though.

I have learned many things from my grandfather, He reminds me constantly not to worry about the petty things in life. This is how it will remain forever. Some people may not agree with the lessons he has taught me. They include: not always respecting my elders, or even not always listening to them, speaking my mind, and not giving a second thought to what people think about me. PawPaw is one of the most important people in my life. No textbook could teach me half the things that I have learned from him already in fifteen years time.

Lauren

At first very tiny, bumping into everything in sight, marvelous balance in precarious situations, totally unseeing on solid ground. My soulmate from day one. How did I know her? Where had we met? She grabbed my heart and has always held it.

What else could I sing to quiet her deep lament at entering a world that she knew would be painful—but limericks. They express in explicit imagery the insanities and ugliness that are present everywhere and encourage thumbing your nose at it and laughing in place of being beaten down.

My life is brightened by every moment I spend with her. We speak the same language without uttering a word. Although the distance between us has grown wider, the bond that unites us is so flexible and strong she is always in my thoughts somewhere.

Today I read some words she wrote about my presence inside of her. She knows me so well— only two mistakes. I am five feet six inches tall and my suits are from 1960.

Lauren is one of the most important people in my life. All of the textbooks I have read over a span of over seventy four years have not come close to teaching me whatI have learned from her in the fifteen and a half years she has been on this planet

For years I had wondered why in the world I had chosen limericks, of all things, as an infant's lullaby. I had no words to explain it until I wrote the essay. What is highlighted for me is how the concept of good enough gives room, and lays the groundwork, for the truth to be fully uncovered and received no matter what is involved. It does not mean that noone's perfect, even though thank goodness that is true. It does mean that so-called perfection fortunately does not exist in human relationships, for if it did the results would be deadly. Thus to have perfection be a goal(even an unattainable one)could only lead one down a false and terrible path.

HEAVEN ON EARTH

My eyes popped open with the first glimpse of sunrise—a new day! I couldn't wait to get up. Here I was two and a half years old feeling eager and ready to meet any new adventure that would arise. For a long time I didn't really understand why this segment of my life stood out in such bold relief. I only knew I could recall it as if it happened yesterday. What did puzzle me were the blank spaces in my memories from either before or afterwards. Much later I was able to recall what my life was like for a six month span of time at age two, and then there was no mystery.

At first there were just fragments that made no real sense. These consisted of flashes of settings, all associated with a nameless feeling of foreboding; no people but a lagoon in a park, a kitchen with an old stove, or a tiny bathroom. When the underlying memories finally pushed their way into the forefront of my mind, it clarified the one thing I did recall. I vividly remembered my thoughts at bedtime, when I would be thinking of what the next day had to bring. Sometimes I would say to myself, "Oh good, it will be a pain day", or "Oh no, it's a terror day". Those weren't exactly the words I used but that was the idea. It seemed like I could manage pain better than fear, and I never attributed much more to the memory. Just the active immagination of a two year old child trying to grasp the world of human emotions.

Once the memories came a lot of things were clarified. I was under the care of a very sadistic woman, babysitting me during the day while my parents were at work. She was very adept at creating painful sensations in all parts of my body without leaving marks, but this was something I could endure. Mostly, I just withdrew deep into myself where I was at one with my bodily processes. The pain being inflicted was primarily on the surface areas and thus was manageable, although I knew even then that I had to make it appear like it was unbearable. The terror, however, was another matter. Being held under the water for long stretches of time was the worst; whether it was over the side of a rowboat in a nearby park lagoon or the inside of a bathtub. This I truly couldn't stand yet I had to somehow. It finally stopped when a neighbor reported what looked to her like suspicious things happening to me. Shortly thereafter we moved to live with with my grandparents and an unmarried aunt and uncle.

Once that took place I knew I was safe and my days were greeted by me with great excitement as a result. Each day started exactly the same way and it was wonderful. My uncle was the first to arise very early and we shared his favorite breakfast; crackers and milk. More importantly we also shared a moment of quiet contact. He was shy with most people, rarely saying much at all, but we had very welcome discussions. This is interesting to me as I look back for they were about baseball. He loved the game, as I do now, and was a catcher on his team. The family couldn't understand what he saw in it as he was often injured (in those days he didn't use a mask, so his nose was broken many times). I'm sure that played a part in how and why I also came to love the game, yet I shake my head as I try to imagine how much I could have understood from ages two and a half to four. Obviously enough for we both enjoyed being together.

My uncle got up, went off to work, and into the kitchen walked my aunt. I loved her dearly. She was peppy, bright, spoke right to the point, and probably most significant laughed at many of the things I would say. Sweet rolls and coffee were her breakfast (orange juice for me), and then she was on her way always a little late. Over the years we remained quite close, and I continued to be able to make her laugh even when she was mad at me for one thing or another.

The real highlight of the morning was my Zadie's appearance. By this time I had been up for quite awhile, though he assumed I was sitting at the table because I was hungry. Teasing me about my huge appetite, which was true even though he didn't know that this was to be my third breakfast, he directed my Baube to be sure and make enough to fill me. While she fixed matzos and eggs he sipped hot tea from a glass. These moments were cherished by me for he would then start talking about his day; the people he would be seeing on his way to schul (his first stop), or the situations he was facing in his work. Whatever topic he would bring up usually elicited short criptic comments from my Baube. His responses were followed by explanations to me, so that I was included in the entire conversation. I was fascinated. Their language with each other was entirely in Yiddish, whereas with me it was mostly English. Nevertheless I came to understand the language fairly well. To this day I can still follow such conversations. Without realizing it I was getting quite an education on how two people can see the circumstance in such different ways. My Zadie was an eternal optimist looking for the best in people. His wife was the opposite, an extreme pessimist searching for the worst. The way they went about it was also interesting. In no way could it be called a fight or argument, since neither insisted that the other agree. It was as if that they each expected the other to see it precisely the way they did.

The remainder of my day was determined solely by me and I enjoyed it enormously. There was no abuse to face or contend with and I was free to travel around the neighborhood. Traffic in those days was minimal so I could easily explore safely, and I indulged in many fantasy games. For example, I had heard much talk about the Lindbergh baby being kidnapped. I would then imagine myself escaping from being discovered by whomever I might see. There was also a small delicatessen a short distance away, where people soon came to recognize me, and I would be invited to taste something they had just prepared.

With the setting sun I would head back, for everyone was returning from work and it was time for dinner. In addition, it was a signal to me to reestablish my relationship with my teddy bear. He had been carefully placed upright in a special chair the moment I woke up. There was no need for him until this particular moment. The activity level in the household escalated as everyone was either preparing the meal or unwinding from whatever their day had brought. What this meant to me was the possibility of orders being given as to what to do (wash your hands), or at some point later when to go to bed. Therefore teddy had to be in place as everyone had been informed that I only took orders from him. They all respected the position he occupied so any directions had to go through him. He was the only one I listened to. In recalling these moments I'm sure I was sensitive to where lines could conceivably be drawn, and teddy undoubtedly was very careful to stay within them. Yet even as I am writing I can feel the hackles rise inside were it to be challenged. I think once I had been freed of the abuse I emerged with what I could only call a vow to never be a victim again. It also feels like it became stronger as I grew older and had access to more options.

It's only now that I'm able to find words for what it felt like at the time. There are a lot of little spin offs, expressed metaphorically, like having one's feet on the ground, feeling at peace with the world, or knowing your heart is in the right place. The experience itself is even more powerful than these descriptions would suggest. It's more like an epiphany; an electric moment of noting integration. Sometimes it takes place at a rapid pace, so it is hard to see exactly what is coming together. At other times the movements are much slower as previously isolated experiences are establishing a connection. The sensation includes the relationship, or relationships, that provided the necessary conditions. Perspective was emerging to aid in enabling my growth. I could feel an acute awareness that emotional connections cannot be maintained without gaps and interruptions. The nature of human communications demands it; it's inevitable, and they are always there. Whenever there are problems in communication, they are the result of someone's fault (most likely all parties concerned), since a fault is a gap. With the emergence of perspective I could also see another person's side so that whatever occurred did not have to be a repetition of earlier traumatic abandonments. The ebb and flow of my own mind could then be observed in awe, regardless of the content and unimpeded by anxiety. Simply stated the environment I had entered fostered this process within me as lightning was transformed into electricity.

I couldn't have been in a better place while the wounds inflicted on my mind and body were healing. In the process of writing this now I can see that a foundation was forming during this period that would serve me well later. Being surrounded by people who made it abundantly clear just how I was affecting them was a vital factor in enabling and supporting the integration that was taking place inside of me. Of course much of this was either wordless or through the vehicle of their own stories. It was in immersing myself in their stories that I was able to discover what was present deep within me. With my uncle it was his baseball stories, my aunt with her delight in hearing whatever I had to say, and my zadie his making sure I would feel a part of his encounters with life.

Throughout my life I had a sense of the potential stories possessed for communicating the impact another person was having upon me. Not that it was the only way, but it made me acutely aware of how significant this kind of knowledge was in facilitating the process of integration. It brought to mind once again what it was like for me in my first encounter with a large group of analysts. Consciously I felt totally intimidated: they seemed so intelligent and filled with profound abstract ideas. At the time I felt so out of place. Therefore when a fellow student greeted me with "do you play baseball?", it was such a relief. Someone knew me. Later he told me why he had asked. He saw me wince as various people spoke(these were the moments when I was consciously feeling intimidated), and his impression was that I was thinking" Isn't there anyone here who grasps what human relationships are all about?" Of course this was what he was consciously thinking. However, his words resonated strongly with what I hadn't been aware of; and I had now found a friend.

Fortunately many others have appreciated how important it is to let someone know the effect they are having if integration is to be properly supported. Certainly throughout history there have been many voices expressing the power such an approach offers in human relationships. It is surprising, therefore, that so frequently psychoanalysts would see it as an interference, and be extremely critical of those who would espouse it.

I often wondered why it was that I had no memory of when I actually left at age four; lots of memories afterwards, but none of the actual separation. It wasn't until much later when I noticed my extreme reaction to the goodbyes to children and grandchildren at moments of parting, that it dawned upon me. I was enacting the unremembered memory of leaving what was truly heaven on earth.

Friends, Allies, And Teachers.

I didn't begin writing until late in my life, and when I did I dedicated my first book in the following fashion: "to my teachers; My family who taught me to love, Missy who taught me about autonomy, Rebel who taught me about life, and my patients who taught me what to write". On several occasions I was asked who Missy and Rebel were and why I had used their nicknames. I guess it was hard to take in that some of my most important teachers have been dogs(literally speaking, that is.). So it is that this book, which has tried to present a picture of my education, would not be complete without adding the part they have played. Over the course of my lifetime there have been many, each having made a contribution, but some had what seemed like special expertise.

Missy was noteworthy in this regard right from the first moment we met her. Our family was ready to receive a new animal member so we began searching in a variety of places. We all knew that this was a serious undertaking, probably as important and unpredictable as adopting a child. We were faced with the challenge of finding an animal that fit in with the emotional climate of our family, yet how best to provide the opportunity for a mutual choice to be made was unclear. The animal has neither the authority nor the words, so it would depend solely on our ability to recognize if and when a choice was made. We saw quite a few puppies, felt drawn to them in one way or another, but the "click" we were looking for just didn't happen. That is; until we came upon a litter of English Setter puppies. One was smaller than the rest, off to the side, bullied by her litter mates and ignored by her mother. The look in this puppy's eyes as she shifted her gaze to each of us, carried a powerful message. It was as if she was appealing to all of us to rescue her. Uncharacteristically(we were told later) she nudged her litter mates aside so she could gain access to our touch. That was it, we just knew there was a proper fit and so it was. There was not even a moment when she whined, cried, or looked unhappy in any way once she joined us. Thus a frisky, energetic, almost human little dog entered our world.

She had an amazing ability to understand directions and constantly showed herself eager to learn our language. Equally striking was how well she communicated her needs to us. In contrast to most other dogs I've known she exhibited no

66

interest whatsoever in anyone outside of our family, tending to back away from many. We found her attributes to be so exceptional that for the first time we decided to allow her to have a litter of puppies. Thus we eagerly awaited the time when she would be in heat, but when it arrived we thought she was still too young. However, we were not prepared for the horde of dogs attracted by her scent. Taking her for walks was an adventure. In the process we became acquainted with every dog in the neighborhood. My children grabbed onto the obvious sexual advances to raise a host of questions, I suspect many of them having been hard to find words for prior to this event. The focus on what was taking place right in front of our noses(so to speak) gave them something to be explicit about, which brought out into the open how it was affecting them. It was also quite a lesson for me, since I tended to find the subject more difficult to talk about than I had realized. It might be stretching it a little, but in looking back I wonder if she wasn't trying to help me in this area. Her responses were so intriguing; from being almost coy, to openly welcoming an approach, to obviously turning away, or at times becoming fearful and untrusting. It all depended upon how sensitive the other dog was to her skittish behavior. It made me think of how she was bullied by her litter mates. Our children's awareness and grasp of sexual matters was certainly furthered by this real life experience, as was my ability to become more comfortable with them.

When being in heat persisted for several weeks we discovered she had an ovarian tumor, leading to the removal of her reproductive organs. Fortunately she recovered quickly and now even more than ever she couldn't tolerate being confined for any length of time. She relished running free in the park and no matter how long we would stay it never seemed to be enough. Clearly she hated a leash as she kept pleading to be given free rein. At first I couldn't grant it, because of all the dangers, especially those associated with traffic. On the other hand I couldn't ignore her persistent appeals. I then spent several weeks working with her around busy streets to see if she could learn to handle cars. It was obvious that she knew what was happening, for once she caught on she became very adept at managing herself even in heavy traffic. Her pride in this accomplishment was touching to see.. A ritual was then established. Late every Saturday night, when traffic was at its lowest ebb, she was let out to be on her own. The next day, usually before dark, she would return with her tongue hanging out in exhaustion—supremely happy…The remainder of the week was no longer a problem, for she was quite content to be on the leash if it was necessary. This concession to her insistence upon a measure of freedom became an integral part of her life.

Then late one Saturday night I received a phone call informing me of her fatal accident. A passer by saw her wanting to cross a street, unaware of her ability to negotiate it. He was worried that she would get hurt and reached out to grab her. She bolted, running right into the path of a car. The loss was particularly painful; first because her life was so short and second because of the irony in how she died. It was an act of kindness, respecting her cry for freedom, that placed her into a position where another act of kindness, trying to assist her, led to her death.

There is an engraved stone I carry with me wherever we live reading, "You brought us your spirit and love of life, thanks big feller". It marks the loss of one of my closest friends, most important allies, and best teacher I have ever had. He was an oversized, dark-orange Golden Retriever, who spent ten unforgettable years with our family. We watched him grow from an awkward, gentle and playful little puppy, confused and bewildered by the world, into a regal appearing, confident, remarkably alert and sensitive dog. His compassionate grasp of non-verbal and even verbal communications grew in ever widening circles. He reminded all of us of Charlie in the story "Flowers for Algernon".

Whenever someone was injured or hurting, he spotted it right away. He would place himself by their side in such a position that the vulnerable area was protected, while his tender loving eyes offered comfort. His greatest pleasure was in chasing and catching squirrels. Proudly placing them at my feet, he paid them little heed as they scampered off unharmed by his soft mouth. He was attuned to who enjoyed feeding or brushing him, who liked active physical play, who got the most out of silent caring involvement, and who simply wanted company at lonely moments. Each member of the family established a distinctly separate relationship on this basis.

The bond of love and trust that had grown between he and I was most clearly shown on a hike our family took in a forest preserve. The area was spotted with a number of small lakes and he had jumped into the water to retrieve a stick. This was his first experience of being in deep water, so we stood at the edge fully expecting him to swim. To our dismay he flailed clumsily trying to stay afloat until he gradually was sinking beneath the water while moving in circles. It suddenly dawned on me that he was drowning. Quick as I could I threw off my clothes and made a flat dive into the water, since I had no idea how deep it was there at the edge. The second I hit the water I knew how silly I was about to look. There was no other recourse but for me to stand up and walk, for I could feel the bottom with my hand and it was only ankle deep for several feet before it dropped off. I wondered, as I swam out to him, how I could carry a panic stricken dog; imagining various positions as I moved closer to where he was. He solved the problem. Just as soon as I got close enough he placed his paws on my shoulders with his head against my neck and he did not move a muscle. The trust he displayed brought tears to my eyes and I swam to shore with him in that position.

After the ordeal was over my family couldn't wait to describe the ridiculous sight of my heroic dive into very shallow water. In spite of the seriousness they could not stop laughing until they saw him mold to my body. It made us all realize how often we take bonds of love and trust for granted and fail to appreciate its power.

Then one fateful day everything changed for him. A booth had been erected for a holiday event in the park right in the middle of his favorite spot. Engaged in his pastime of chasing squirrels he pulled up short to avoid this unexpected obstacle. The resulting stress ruptured two vertebral discs and severed his spinal cord. At first he was totally paralyzed from the spinal shock, but gradually recovered functions in the upper parts of his body. It was agonizing to see his shame at the loss of bowel and bladder control, and his painful unsuccessful attempts to gain mobility. After a thorough examination we were told that he would never walk again, and advised to put him to sleep. I could only say that such a decision rested with him, and I would wait until I had his answer. The looks I received were familiar, for many people believe the idea of communicating with animals is a figment of one's immagination and thus has no validity.

Initially it was hard to tell exactly where he stood. Finally one day, while I was painting a fence, his decision became clearly evident to me. Watching him dragging himself along side of me, his spirit and desire to live was bubbling over at what could only be described as a smile. We spoke without words for some time and as we did my attention was drawn to some faint muscle twitching in his lower body and limbs. My heart leapt and at that moment we made a pact together. I began a daily regimen of exercises designed to work with the thin strands of muscle tissue still having some viability.

Every morning I awoke to find him eagerly waiting to begin. When his legs and lower body developed a little more strength I tried to show him how to walk again. One part of the routine made it necessary for me to bend over in order to support his hind legs as I moved them forward. It hurt my back, so I could only sustain it for short segments of time, but I kept doing it because it seemed promising. I'll never forget the morning I knew that he would succeed. There I was struggling to move his leg when I happened to look up and see him smiling at me. I had the distinct impression he was holding back his ability to walk in order to playfully tease me. It was an exhilarating moment for me, the first indication

I'd had that there might be any hope. Sure enough one week later he maneuvered on his own. It could hardly have been called walking as he was clumsy and could only manage a few steps. Gradually, however, he became more adept. There were occasional setbacks, especially in wintry weather, but he quickly recovered. Now he chased frogs instead of squirrels.

The lessons he taught about courage, determination, pride, and loving involvement have never been forgotten. In addition he taught my son a profound lession about the meaning of compassion. It played a significant roll in guiding his way into a medical career, and probably was a major factor in his acceptance into medical school. At the time of the accident my son couldn't tolerate the anguish he experienced at seeing his friend so debilitated. He either tearfully pitied him or avoided contact. Whenever this proud animal was in my son's company, he would behave like a helpless invalid. It took my son awhile to see the destructive impact his attitude was having. When he did it opened his eyes to how much his personal reactions were hurting a highly valued relationship. The two of them were then able to reestablish their playful connection. When he applied to medical school he wrote a letter of reference from his dog. In it he described how they had discovered together the importance of facing injury and illness with an attitude of respect for life, which unleashed the healing power of genuine hope. The consequence was in my son's desire to alleviate suffering becoming more solidified. In his final interview in applying to medical school, just as it was ending, he was asked about his dog seemingly as an after thought. My son is convinced that he was accepted as a result of having that opportunity to explain the circumstances and his reactions to them.

At the age of ten our friend, ally, and teacher developed a brain tumor. His final days were a nightmare consisting of numerous seizures, loss of coordination and balance, and finally his eyesight. When he stopped eating and was in obvious pain, it was evident to everyone but me that he was making an appeal for us to help him die with dignity. During his final hours, as I was holding him, he tried in vain to eat something. His inability to do so helped me to see that he was ready and I was having trouble letting him go. Our family then gathered together to say our goodbyes. When the veternarian came to our house to put him to sleep he died quietly after lifting his head to look deeply into my eyes.

Without a word being spoken my son and I built a coffin, dug a grave, and buried him in our backyard. Afterwards we all missed him. In reminiscing about the place he occupied in each of our lives, we became aware of how he had managed to have special moments at different times of the day or night, so that one or another of us was with him practically around the clock. My son and I were also struck by what we had done. Usually neither one of us can locate anything we are looking for and are all thumbs when it comes to handling tools. Incredible what a meaningful relationship is capable of bringing out.

There have been some animals who are a joy to watch as they do what appears to be teaching, although it's probably impossible to know if that is their intent. A good example of this was shown in a lesson three granddaughters received from an excellent teacher. He was a large, black Australian shepherd with a long bushy tail and a loud penetrating bark. He had been my son's companion during his medical school years and was temporarily in our care until they could be reunited after his internship. His exclusive attachment was to my son, which was apparent in a constant search for his return. On one occasion an exact replica of my son's car drove down our street and he ran out excitedly to greet him. Immediately noting that it was another person he became very depressed and wouldn't eat for several days. However, he did feel comfortable with us. In living with him we were struck by his gentle sensitive nature, which was in constrast to an outward appearance of being somewhat wild and possibly ferocious. The ease with which he followed directions was also noteworthy, as was his strong desire to please. He always tried to understand what was being asked of him. Nevertheless my granddaughters were terrified whenever they came close to him; reacting as though he was a frightening monster.

Children who have had little direct contact with animals will tend to see them as having a life much like their own. When the animal seemingly behaves differently it can make them appear to be a threat. Therefore getting to know and understand an animal can go far in helping a child to see beyond the surface appearances of its behavior. There is then a real chance to discover that what initially may be terrifying can be looked into more deeply and turn out to be a friend. It's not always an easy task to know when and how to negotiate the first step. This dog, however, led the way and his teaching methods were fascinating to observe. First, and probably foremost, he approached them gently letting them know he was interested. Then he just patiently waited for them to be comfortable, while silently demonstrating his readiness to receive directions. They were impressed by how much he understood and took great pleasure in telling him what to do and watching him comply. Soon he searched for, and found, a ball to engage them in play. In short order they came to enjoy being with him. It was not surprising that their fear of other animals, as well as unfamiliar children, also dissipated.

The time came for him to return to my son and plans were made to drive him there. His apparent realization of what was happening was astounding. Several days prior to leaving he began trying to crawl into the back of the car at every opportunity, sitting there contentedly as though he was ready to go. On one occasion he had jumped through an open car window, so we didn't know where he was for several hours, until we came upon him calmly waiting. By this time my granddaughters had become very fond of him. They felt very sad about his going away, but they could also see how much it meant to him. Their farewell was heart warming. Each gave him a big hug, waving a little tearfully as the car pulled away. That moment captured how much they had learned and what a good teacher he had been.

Certainly the non-verbal aspects of human communication are well known; still there is a remarkable tendency to overlook there influence on our every day life. A great deal is expressed through body language, tone of voice, and other unspoken gestures. These subtle messages are constantly being picked up and reacted to without specifically noticing their source. What is done usually has more meaning and a greater impact than what is said, while communication flows when words and behavior match. Relationships with animals, and in this regard with infants as well, furnish a constant reminder of the significance of these non-verbal exchanges. In addition, their very presence is a marvelous antidote for the dehumanizing elements that invade a person's life. The nature of an animal's being does not allow materialistic concerns to be a factor in the attachment. Instead treasured qualities of loyalty, trust, involvement, and love are highlighted. What better way is there to keep the priorities, giving depth and meaning to life, more clearly in focus.

MY FAILURE DINNER

Seemingly out of the blue I received a phone call from a second cousin I had not seen for years. I had known her quite well as a child, and maintained contact even after I was married. From that point our lives had gone in different directions. Her son was planning to attend college in our city and she was worried about his being in a strange and unfamiliar place. She remembered how well he and I had gotten along when he was a toddler, so she thought it would be helpful if he knew someone near by were any trouble to arise. He and I then spoke briefly in order to arrange a meeting place and had fun imagining what each of us could wear to make sure we would find each other. Finally we decided to just go there and see what would happen.

I recognized him immediately, for though he had grown tall his features remained the same. To my surprise he also recognized me. Our playful interactions that had started when he was small, had continued just a little bit on the telephone, now quickly came alive as we met in person. It did not take long for him to become incorporated into our family. Initially, he was somewhat stiff and formal, having been raised in a very strict home where being polite and proper was emphasized. Our children loved to joke around with him, as he did with them, and his outward appearance of aloofness faded away as he dropped this facade.

He had a life long dream of becoming a doctor, which he had pursued despite pressure from his family to move in other directions. Throughout his school years he had always made top grades and he continued this same pattern in his pre-med courses. These grades were incredibly important to him and he worked very hard to make sure he never even received a B. We all shared in his excitement the day he was accepted into medical school. The high hopes he felt as he entered were diminished somewhat when he was overwhelmed by the vast amount of material he had to learn. He had not yet discovered that this was simply par for the course, since no human being could possibly master all that was presented. Never having confronted such a situation he was thrown for a loop, and he even began to question his ability. Having the idea that this was probably a good lesson for him, plus knowing how well he had done to get this far, we teased him a lot about his

uncertainty. Now he was approaching his first examination with great trepida-
tion.

So it was that we were all caught off balance when he walked in one day, after
the results came in, looking totally shattered and distraught. He had flunked the
exam! This was the first time he had ever experienced a failure in anything, which
filled him with despair about the likihood of ever realizing his dream. Upon this
background a tradition was born. We called it a failure dinner.

The event itself was memorable; each of us toasted his failure in a satirical and
humorous way. We used every adjective we could think of to applaud his remarkable achievement. We then insisted that he takea bow. With that gesture he
joined in the spirit of the occasion. He proceeded to give a speech thanking us for
celebrating this successful failure with him. The light in his eyes as he spoke
showed that he had gotten the message; that is, to keep his yearning and striving
for what was meaningful alive without compromising what he knew to be true
within himself. Without directly expressing it in words we were all encouraging,
in him and in ourselves, belief in the impossible. This failure dinner was designed
to highlight the value of a total passionate investment in a cherished goal, with
the actual result being secondary to the value of the effort and the experience.

The idea had arisen spontaneously as a way of giving comfort to the devastation he felt in failing the exam. It was also giving him credit for the effort he put
in. The hope was that he would learn from the experience, instead of being
defeated, so he could the place the failure in proper perspective. In fact it accom-
plished much more than we could have imagined. The power of what had
occurred had an impact on all of us. It remains to this day as a part of our families
system of values. Thus a failure dinner is prescribed for any family member falling down on the pathway towards reaching an impossible dream.

In order to be eligible one has to become completely involved in attaining a
personally desired venture, and then either stumble along the way or actually fail.
The purpose is to honor the willingness to put everything into it without regard
as to the outcome. Then support can be given to following what is in one's heart
even though on the surface it may seem to be unrealistic. Hopefully it can fuel
any remaining incentive to try once again, irrespective of the obstacles.

During the course of my professional life I harbored a secret dream, waiting
for the time and opportunity to try and bring it into fruition. Over the years psychiatric settings that I had come in contact with were losing their humanistic
concerns. They had become infused with the priorities of materialistic consider-
ations and externally mandated standards. I had hoped to build a healing environment accessible to anyone who could make use of it, manned by people

dedicated to a love of the truthand capable of providing sensitive psychological care. I pictured it including a residential setting,wherein the unique treatment needs of a given individual could be met around the clock; a school, tailored to the special educational needs of children unable to find it elsewhere; and an out patient clinic for those whose growth was best facilitated while they were engaged in their daily lives. It was a dream that became more elaborate with each passing year, and as I gained more experience what I learned was incorporated in it.

In my fantasies, for example, there was some version of the "Southard School" refrigerator. This was a residential setting for children that had a well stocked refrigerator right smack in the middle of the living room. One staff members assignment was to keep it constantly filled with a variety of healthy foods of all kinds. The purpose was to communicate a non-verbal message that every effort would be exerted to provide nourishment for growth. There were no restrictions and anyone could help themselves to their heart's desire. At first I had a negative reaction thinking it could also feed greedy strivings, as well as unhealthy collusions. To my surprise almost all of the children followed a similar pattern of behavior; initial disbelief, followed by testing of its reality by hoarding and accumulating huge quantities in hidden places, and then relaxing to enjoy the availability. In those few instances where it did feed unhealthy strivings it brought them out into the open where they could be discussed not simply prohibited. I came to like and value that idea. Another example concerns the locks on mental hospital doors. This one made complete sense to me. I had never really understood the concept behind a patient being locked up. Oh, I knew there were many patients who felt safer that way, and many staff people who were fearful of not having that control. Most frequently it looked to me like a substitute for adequate care. In my opinion the locks should be on the inside so a patient has control over who is let in, rather than on the outside so others control whether the patient is let out.

When my youngest child went off to college I decided the time was right to translate my dream into reality. I didn't think it would be supported in the city I lived in, so I began to search for other locales. There were a number of places that expressed interest in what I was proposing, but upon exploring them further none of them would grant the level of autonomy I insisted upon. One group met with me and were intrigued by my ideas. When it came to the point of defining the specifics they initiated the discussion by stating I had to agree to work thirty-five hours per week. I simply responded that there could be no conditions of that nature. In explanation, I tried to get across to them how the nature of this work required an honest assesstment by each individual of what they could do in order to be fully there. External demands could not be a determining factor. I did not mention that thirty-five hours per week was usually too short a work week for me, for it was irrelevant to my point. It became vividly apparent that they had no concept of what I meant by autonomy, until I finally found a way to make it unmistakeable. I asked if I would have the authority to hire and fire people. They assured me of that and realized its importance. I then raised a hypothetical situation where we agreed on what path was right to take, but for whatever reason disagreed on whether it would be feasible. In addition we found it was impossible to reconcile our differences. I then wondered if under those circumstances I could fire them. The answer was obvious and our discussion was over. I met with this same impasse everywhere I looked.

Another large institution was quite interested in the possibility of developing my ideas as a research project. The thesis would be to see if effective treatment could be done on a more limited budget and thus be free of the restrictions imposed by outside agencies. I had already indicated my observation that most treatment centers were highly overbudgeted, by virtue of the way they distributed and financed care. Many in this group knew me and they spent six months going back and forth as to whether they would support it. Finally a decision was made to turn it down with the statement, "we know how important autonomy is, and we try to encourage it as much as possible, but he would really expect it". They were quite right Now the decision was totally in my hands.

In spite of my suspicion that my community would not be open to supporting such a venture, I went ahead. First I let it be known that I was starting a new facility. I interviewed people to select a staff, rented and renovated an old house to serve as the setting, and sent out announcements. The doors of what was called The Growth Center were then opened. Starting out on a small scale, it operated essentially as an patient clinic. There was a one room school for a very limited number of children, which we were hoping to gradually expand. In the background plans were present to move towards providing overall care.

The first task was to take what ever steps were necessary to ensure that sound treatment principles would reign supreme. Because we required outside financial support I knew that this meant having a board of directors. I also thought, from previous experience, that the relationship between boards and clinicians were completely backwards. Usually the clinician was responsible to the board, which seemed to me to be inappropriate and unfair to both parties—a complete misuse of their knowledge and expertise. It only made sense to me to have the board responsible to the clinician. I was to find out later that this made fund raising impossible. Nevertheless I found a new firm who worked several months (pro-bono thank goodness) to find enough loop holes so as to make it legally feasible.

The budding organization then seemed to be getting off of the ground. Unnecessary red tape was eliminated, the working conditions were designed to protect and foster the autonomous functioning of therapists, and teaching and learning were an integral part of each day. In addition outside consultants were brought in periodically to serve as a stimulus to new ideas. These were primarily old friends who were pleased to help out. They were exciting days. My time, day and night, was occupied with seeing patients, teaching, and meeting with members of the community to acquaint them with what we were doing and seek their support.

I quickly discovered that in the arena of administrative functions like establishing a board and raising funds I was a total disaster. This was an entirely new and foreign world to me; I didn't understand the language and I was much too naive concerning the unspoken rules that dictated so-called proper behavior. My efforts to call this to everyones attention were basically ignored, especially by those people who had volunteered to serve on the board. So there I was, hung out to dry, doing the best I could, which was not very good.

Several examples illustrate the problem I was having. The members of the board were all people who had been informed of our undertaking by members of the staff, and had listened to my description of what we were attempting to do. Supposedly out of their wish to support what they considered a worthly organization they volunteered their services. They would guide me as to who to talk to and even arrange meetings where I would make a presentation in order to gain financial support. I never understood what the actual board meetings were all about. I tried on several occasions to give an overview, with examples, of the nature of our work. This did not appear to be very welcome. Finally I was told in private by one of the members that I was remiss. My task was to make everyone feel important. Thus I was directed to arrange separate times to speak with each member where I could do something akin to what I was doing with the group. The board meetings were a place for them to form policies of accountability, which basically meant to put in place all of the things I had eliminated as red tape, or worse things that compromised a therapist's autonomy. Whenever I attempted to bring this out in the open for discussion, I was met with annoyance. Another board member, who had just sold his company and could have easily provided the entire amount we required to put the complete package in place, took me aside to "set me straight". He went into a lengthy description of his younger years, placing emphasis upon his idealistic approach to his life. Very quickly he learned that he had to compromise his ideals if he was to be successful, and so he did. There was no way then that he would provide me the means to succeed under the idealistic principles I was espousing. It was important to him that I too compromise, and when he saw me doing that the financial support would follow.

I was also having difficulty in dealing with my reactions to what I faced in meeting with philanthropic groups. It all came to a head one day after a series of several meetings that week. My appointment was with the director of a large organization that assessed the merits of non-profit enterprises. It was the middle of the day, a busy time for me, so I came in having had to rush to get there. He came into the waiting room just as I arrived and indicated where I could sit. Pausing for a moment he looked up and asked "so, tell me what it is that makes what you are doing unique?" I really find it hard to know exactly what hit me, for I found myself getting up to leave as I said "I think that's a great question, but I'm so f——ing sick of answering it I'm out the door", and away I went. I could hardly believe what I had said and done, but it was a clear message that from that moment on someone else would have to do it. It just couldn't be me.

This was the beginning of the end, though The Growth Center did go on awhile longer. In all it lasted for seven years. I had simply had it with all the double talk, the demands for conformity, and the insistance on what was called accountability. We, in fact, were much more accountable than any of the procedures would have ensured. I saw other organizations gain large amounts of funding by just outright lying. It was, as they said, standard operating procedure. Everyone wanted to know what the matter was with me. That's how it worked. You found out what was expedient to say and you said it. Then there was the yes-no phenomena. This was the unspoken rule that you never put a philanthropist in the position of having to say no. Answers such as "we have met our quota this month, come back in January", meant no, and so you were to let it be. I would return in January only to be told it was March, and if I came in March it was June. Finally a call was made to make sure I was informed of that rule. There was also the "girl scout cookie"message. This was a specified amount, not too big or small, that meant "we'll do it once as a favor to a friend, but then forget it". All of the duplicity, hypocrisy, and double messages left me in a whirl. At one point I was asked how I could go back to work with patients right after spending time in a sequence of these exhausting meetings. I laughed, because I couldn't wait until I was doing just that. During this period it was the sanest experience I was having.

The Growth Center thus represented the realization of my impossible dream. I had devoted all of the energy I possessed into trying to make it a viable institution. After a promising start it became evident that it could not exist in the way I visualized without extensive backing. What was needed would clearly not be forthcoming, and I did not have the kind of personality traits that could make it work. Therefore The Growth Center finally closed its doors after an interesting life.

With the closure I had met all of the criteria for being the recipient of a failure dinner. I now had first hand knowledge of what it meant to become completely immersed in moving towards realizing a dream and then having that dream collapse. My absorption in reaching for this cherished goal has expanded my understanding of myself, of the world, and of the part I can play in giving meaning to my life. At the dinner itself I also felt the importance of sharing the experience with those I cared about, as they joined me in the celebration. The dinner went far in easing the pain of this successful failure. I could see clearly that chasing rainbows,or believing in miracles,were not necessarily ways of avoiding reality. The entire episode had been a vital journey of discovery. I was finding my unique place in the world, and as a result my resolve to put what I had learned to good use was strengthened.

THE FALL OF CAMELOT

When the letter arrived I had to read it over at least three times to make sure I was taking its message in accurately. It announced an impending move of the setting in which I received my training; that part I had heard rumblings about so I was not at all surprised. What I could hardly believe was the detailed description of all the reasons this would be the most exciting event in the history of psychiatric treatment, training, education, and research. I perceived it as the total and final capitulation to the kind of compromises that had slowly destroyed an institution once devoted to the search for truth. Like every institution there might have been instances of deviating from what was clearly right, but unlike most these were sought out to be exposed, learned from, and discarded. Over the years I had watched the gradual erosion of these principles of integrity, replaced by an elitist attitude that closed the doors to even recognizing what was happening. It was sad to see, for the years I spent there were so deeply valued by me. Thus the tone of the announcement of its demise, under the pretense of it being a cause for celebration, vividly captured what had been lost.

The letter also announced that there would be a reunion of alumni to honor this momentous decision. A session was set aside for various people to present their view of what the setting meant to them, as a way of launching this new and exciting development. I just shook my head, and then wondered if there might be any remnant of openness to hearing a conflicting point of view. I thought of the years I had spent there and how at that time such opportunities were sought. People whose ideas were at odds with cherished concepts were often invited to both speak and participate. This was considered to be a challenge and an opportunity to expand our vision, or to incorporate something that had been overlooked. The tenor of the letter, as well as the slow erosion of welcoming ideas that could place the setting in a bad light, suggested that what I had to say would not only be unwelcome but also not allowed.

My thoughts drifted back to the tremendous spur to learning so many visitors brought. I recalled a short conversation with Helen Keller, after her lecture, which made a big impact on me. We "spoke" through her interpreter. What amazed me was her ability to establish a strong emotional connection to a complete stranger (me), and communicate it without being able to "see" or "hear" me. My eyes were opened to the power of non-verbal communication.

In the same vein a famous, or more accurately infamous, psychiatrist came to demonstrate his "technique" for "curing" schizophrenia. He asked that he be given a very sick individual and he would cure him during the ten day period of his visit. The sessions were conducted behind a two-way mirror. Twenty four hours of every day, only interrupted by short periods of sleep, were spent interacting with the patient. This patient had not spoken to anyone for years, occupying himself by crawling along the floor chewing on the wood work. At the end of the ten days there was no doubt that the patient was not cured, but there also was no doubt that he had been reached. In observing what this doctor did, it looked as though he simply insisted that everything had meaning and he was going to discover it no matter what. After awhile the patient stopped crawling around the floor and began to interact verbally, even though it was hard to grasp what he was saying. That scenario, however, made me wonder about applying it to a group of patients that were a terrible problem at the time. These were people diagnosed as being in a state of catatonic excitement, which if not interrupted was life threatening. They would literally be climbing the walls non stop until they perished if it was not stopped. The only answer seemed to be electric shock treatment, which worked, but to me seemed like an awful way to treat another human being. Therefore, when the next occasion arose, I put on old clothes and basically adopted the same posture in interacting with a patient. Sometimes I could just sit and comment on the meaning of the patient's kicking and screaming, though at other times I had to physically intervene to prevent the patient or myself from getting hurt. This went on for a long time, probably three or four hours, yet lo and behold the patient settled down. The acute episode was over. No EST! Others who tried this also found that it was successful. In examining the times that it was not, much seemed to depend upon whether the doctor was able to put his or her heart and soul into it. This was quite a lesson.

Another example involved a world reknowned neuropsychiatrist, whose ideas about mental illness were strictly related to the functioning of the brain to the exclusion of emotional factors. She was especially known for her expertise with autistic children. At the time of her visit we were having difficulty establishing an accurate diagnosis with a very young child who was suspected of showing early signs of autism. An interview was scheduled in front of a two way mirror and she bustled in somewhat late, settling back in a chair to observe. Sitting right next to her I noted that she promptly fell sound asleep. The interview ended, the lights were turned on, and she proceeded to discuss the case. To my amazement she gave a very lucid account of the child's trouble from her perspective, outlining the various disturbed brain functions that were manifested in his behavior. Although I realized she had not really seen this child, her discussion did shed light on some aspects of his behavior. It helped a lot in broadening my understanding of the mind as a part of the body, not some separate entity as I tended to believe.

Meanwhile I began to feel an urge to express my feelings at the reunion, unwanted though they might be, as I suspected I wasn't alone. I thought the least I could do was to give an honest appraisal of what I considered to be a funeral and thus say good-bye to a cherished institution. I knew the person in charge of the program and, while I was composing a letter to him, memories of my training days came flooding back. Little snippets here and there that said so much.

At one point a few residents (myself included) volunteered to work with groups of delinquent children at a local boys reform school. We all quickly realized we didn't know any thing about what we were doing. We asked for supervision, but after a few days when we hadn't received an answer we just knew exactly what to do. There was a weekly news letter published, which had a small section reserved for any announcements of special events. We placed an ad stating that there was to be a meeting of the "residents who couldn't find supervision" club at seven p.m. on Thursday night. The news letter was distributed on a Tuesday and we were informed the following day that Dr. F. would be there to lead the discussion. He was a very well known figure who had studied under August Aichorn (famous for his work with delinquent children). This incident showed the high priority given to providing support and teaching for any interest that permeated the atmosphere. The idea of someone wanting such help and not being able to find it was unthinkable. The seminar itself was great, as you might imagine, since all of its members were so highly motivated.

In that same context when I realized that I would have to leave after my final year of training (we had to find special education for one of my children), I dealt with it by finding eight different supervisors. I knew I needed to learn much more to have any degree of competence. With this in mind first I selected a very knowledgeable, sensitive authority on psychoanalytic thinking, who was adept at translating complex intellectual ideas as they applied to actual experiences. Invaluable. Much later I returned to consult with him about a problem I was having in my position as director of training. While I was trying to get my concern across that I was turning down applicants inappropriately, worried that I was idealizing certain qualities to the point of their being unrealistic. I couldn't help but notice his smile as I talked. It made me think for a moment that he either didn't know or take seriously what I was saying. When I stopped to tell him that, he became serious and explained his smile. My particular group were considered quite unusual in possessing these qualities. In addition we had arrived at a time that he referred to as the Camelot days. The conditions weren't that way before and haven't been since.

The next one I selected was very meticulous, probably to a fault, but I received a good sense of the many things that had to be taken into account and of the dangers of complacency. Next I sought a very wise woman, who had helped me several times in limited consultations. She was reluctant at first, for she had never supervised anyone before, but finally agreed. Later she told me that she had stayed away from this area because of her distrust of doctors. What she found most surprising in me was how aware I was of not knowing anything. After, and even during, our supervisory work we became good friends. Another was an assignment not a choice. This was a person who had spent many years as a naval officer, and his organizational, administrative skills were a big asset. I had a lot to learn in that arena, and he had a lot to teach. It was a good match for there was absolutely no pretense that he had anything to offer that extended into other areas.

The others had more to do with my desire to take advantage of the expertise of some very special people while I still could. One was a psychologist whose ability to use and interpret tests seemed quite striking to me. I had sat in on many conferences where the results of such tests were read, but my knowledge of how such information could be derived was quite limited and even more I had no sense as to whether the interpretations were accurate. Therefore I arranged regular meetings to in essence take a course so I would be capable of assessing what I was hearing. In that regard as I was engaged in that effort I paid particular attention to another psychologist who appeared equally as knowledgeable. His reports were read in a very sophisticated and professional fashion, sounding like he had spent a great deal of time in preparing them. On one occasion I happened to be sitting next to him and he mentioned something I wasn't sure of, so I leaned over to read it from the paper he was holding. It was totally blank! What a talent. It turned out he was way behind on his reports and thus presented it in this way. It cracked me up and my reaction made it hard for him to continue as he was choking back his own laughter. This was my introduction to what became a good friendship.

Another was a social worker who had the most sensitive, empathic grasp of even the most complex family dynamics that I ever encountered. Furthermore his down to earth manner in expressing these insights was even more impressive. Added to that was a wonderful sense of humor, which made him a gifted teacher.

Quite an important figure for the budding child psychiatrist I was at the time. Then there was a quiet, very laid back neurologist, who was fascinated with the task of unravelling mind-body connections, and of identifying the behavioral evidence of brain malfunctioning. I just knew this was something I had to learn more about, and so he made time available to me. Finally, there was an aging child psychiatrist, nearing his retirement, who no longer saw patients but spent his time consulting with schools. The wealth of practical information that he possessed was mind boggling and it was a treat to listen to him talk. He clearly enjoyed spending time with me, using my experiences in consulting with a local school as an excuse to just talk together about people in general and institutions in particular. He got a kick out of my tendency to be rebellious (I think it matched his own), but would offer creative solutions that weren't as abrasive as mine. Clearly I enjoyed these moments with him.

In retrospect I think the first cracks in the structure of the setting were beginning to show the year before I actually left. One of the most revered teachers came in conflict with the head of the organization over some matter of the curiculum he was to teach. Because it couldn't be resolved without that teacher relinquishing his autonomy, he opted to leave. I did not know him at all but would have chosen him as a supervisor if it had been possible. Thus I felt sad both about the reasons for his leaving and for missing an opportunity to get to know and learn from him. On the eve of his departure he gave a seminar devoted to fairy tales. I was absolutely captivated by his presentation. He alternately read a portion of the fairy tale,which he followed by interpreting its symbolic meaning. What really brought it to life was the passionate way he was immersed in the experience. Amazingly our paths did cross some years later, I did get to know him, and it was my good fortune that we became friends. It occurred when he was invited to speak at a convention held in the city where I had moved. I saw him walking in the halls and walked up to introduce myself. I wanted to tell him how meaningful his discussion of fairy tales had been to me. Before I could say a word he stopped me, closed his eyes for a moment of intense concentration, and then identified the row and seat I was sitting in that final night. He laughed at my shocked reaction and explained. He had noticed that only three people in the audience seemed to be emotionally affected by his words. In order to be fully involved himself he had to concentrate his attention on the three of us, so that when I came close he immediately recognized my face. Needless to say from that point on we discovered we had much in common.

Leaving was extremely hard, not only for me but for my entire family. In looking back I would have had to leave in another two or three years anyway, due to the changes that were taking place. Most of the other attractions of the setting centered around the many close friendships we were forming. Our neighborhood was largely composed of psychiatric colleagues and their families, so that for the children it was like a commune. They just loved the ambiance of being welcomed without any ceremony in so many homes. After we had moved my daughter's first grade teacher asked her class if they could inform everyone of what their fathers did. My daughter immediately thought her teacher must be pretty stupid, for everyone knew that all fathers were psychiatrists.

The more I remembered of the Camelot days the sadder I became. I would have loved the move the organization was making if it was as portrayed in the letter. Over the years I had observed its gradual decline, yet was always hoping that the islands of integrity that remained could rise again. Here now might be a last chance, but there was no indication of anyone speaking out. I knew I was not alone. The person in charge of the reunion was someone I liked and respected, and I also thought would be acutely aware of what had been lost. Therefore I decided to write and request an opportunity to be on the program so I could present my point of view. It was the only way I could picture myself attending and I did want to do that.

Shortly thereafter I received a reply stating that I could not be on the program. He gave a long explanation of why it had been necessary to make the compromises I had referred to. As an addendum he mentioned that I could express my observations in a short question and answer period following the formal presentations. This reply felt to me like the announcement of the death of a very close friend. The apparent lack of openness in a person I had once thought of quite differently was also disappointing.

The following is an edited copy of the letter I wrote in response (leaving names out), which expresses my view of the final fall of Camelot:

Dear X:

Thank you for your thoughtful reply to my letter. I did not go into detail in my short note, so you could not have appreciated either the source or depth of my feeling. In addition my reactions may very well be overdetermined because of the personal situations they involved, while on the other hand your having spent a life time working there may create some blind spots. I will just mention three situations that are symbolic to me of the gradual deterioration I have witnessed in both the quality of care and a slow erosion of integrity that has taken place over the years. At the same time a kind of elitist attitude has emerged to fill in the gaps.

The first instance concerned my daughter who was seriously misdiagnosed, leading to grossly insensitive treatment. Such things are inevitable, though it was not so much the fact that it occurred but the closed minded response to even considering that there was a mistake. It broke my heart at the time, mostly due to the suffering it created for her. In addition, however, my feeling was accentuated by the shattering of my belief in the organization. Fortunately she was able to find what she needed elsewhere and it has made an enormous difference in her life.

The second instance concerns a time when I was establishing the Growth Center (a psychiatric clinic based on my version of idealistic principles nourished during my years of training). We had week-end seminars periodically and Dr. Y was recommended as an expert in schizophrenia (we had a number of such patients). It was a painful experience for everyone, especially him. As you know he was thought of in your organization as an expert in this area. In fact his knowledge was extremely limited, his grasp of dealing with such patients faulty, and he had no concept whatsoever of the problems or necessary approaches in treating very sick people on an outpatient basis. All of that would not have been so bad except for his attitude. To his credit he knew he was in over his head, but he simply refused to consider that it was a grievous error to not distinguish between those who needed a hospital and those for whom it was destructive.

The third is the most serious in regard to my desire to speak. This one has to do with my soulmate and dearest friend, Z. He was such a decent, principled man. Once he was in the position of being director of the hospital it put the very essence of who and what he was in a constant unyielding struggle. Pressure was continually exerted upon him to violate his beliefs, along with many "logical" explanations as to the reasons it had to be done. Many of these rational-lies were along the lines that you mentioned in your letter. Sadly for him he sometimes engaged in such thinking himself. Soon he would be swept up in justifying what was unjustifiable(to him). It literally "broke his heart"(he knew it contributed to his heart attack). My knowledge of the specifics came from our frequent talks. I like to believe I was helpful to him, perhaps, I don't know. During one period of time, as you may or may not know, we spoke almost every day for a year (much of it centering around his work with an extremely sick patient).

Well, at any rate, I think you get the point. Of course the organization had to deal with the destructive impact of managed care(don't we all). I never thought, and still don't, that it had to do with mismanagement of funds as you suggest. Rather, I believe it had to do with an ongoing erosion of principles, so that decisions were made from a whole different foundation than the one I knew and loved. Differences of opinion were exciting challenges not problems, and the common devotion to, and love of, the truth was the compass determining what was done. What happened to that? Sure Z's difficulty was his own doing, just as my reactions are a product of whatever influences have shaped my life. Therefore it is not at all surprising to me that the move would be made. What surprises and disappoints me is that it is given such noble motives with no room for an opposing view. Even if the motive is positive, there clearly is another side that is not being openly addressed. Consequently it seems inevitable to me that the decision to move will ultimately extinguish the fires that once burned brightly. That is what I meant by stating I appreciate and value what it was, and am saddened by what it has become.

I hope this explains my position and I do have an idea of how you must feel. I now have a decision to make and will think about it. There is some reluctance in me to speak under the conditions you mentioned, because of the implication(perhaps unwarranted)that there is not a genuine openness to any opposing point of view. I, in no way, consider myself an oracle of what constitutes the truth, only a person troubled by what appears to be the demise of what a revered organization has always stood for.

Shortly after the reunion it was announced that all plans for the move were scrapped. The reasons for this dramatic, last minute change were left in the dark. The only explanation given was that it had to be kept confidential, as though that displayed a high level of honesty and integrity. Perhaps in someone's mind it did. What took it's place was a proudly stated declaration that another even more advantageous alliance was being sought. Thus it was openly and formally stated that the truth had to be hidden. It could not have been made more evident that although the cherished name would still be retained, the principles upon which it was built had indeed perished.

HYPNOSIS

✦

(How Can Something So Wrong Be Right)

I was fifteen years old, working at a summer camp, when I was first introduced to hypnosis. An older counselor entertained us in the evenings by putting on a show, which totally captured my interest and curiosity. Up to that point I thought of hypnosis as a production of the movies, hardly real, but a means of creating mystery and suspense in horror films. The vision was of some evil satanic person putting an unsuspecting victim under his spell by somehow getting him or her to focus attention on a pendulum swaying back and forth. Even though I thought of it as unreal, I did wonder why it was such an effective vehicle for stirring up fearful feelings. Once I saw this counselor perform there was no doubt as to how real it was.

He usually began by selecting a volunteer to whom he gave an object to concentrate upon. Meanwhile he mumbled repetitively in a monotone directing the person to move deeper into sleep. At some moment, unrecognizable to me at first, he then indicated the person was now hypnotized. Initially my impression was that it all was just an act. However that impression quickly dissolved as he proceeded to have the person doing things such as devouring a raw onion with great relish, after having been told how very thirsty he or she was, before being presented with what was called a delicious orange. Even more striking was to see him place a person with their stiffened body stretched out between two chairs, the top of their head on the back of one and the heel of their foot on the back of the other. At this point someone else would actually stand on the person's suspended body. Afterwards I spent considerable time with him learning this amazing technique. Much to my surprise it turned out to be very easy to accomplish.

He taught me a variety of body reactions to elicit and exploit in order to create the illusion of having control. Gradually this would lead to the individual relinquishing their decision making to the hypnotist. Once that occurs the process is well underway and the level of induction can then spread and deepen. The key factor rested in the confidence of the hypnotist, everything else was simply window dressing to strengthen the aura of mystery. It only took one occasion of being successful in inducing a hynotic trance to have that sense of confidence. At this young age I had no sense whatsoever of anything destructive or hurtful in the procedure; my awareness of that only emerged later. I blithely demonstrated the phenomenon in many situations and I have to admit one primary motive had to do with the attention I received. This was amplified by my fascination with the workings of the human mind and the realization of how much power it had. A number of experiences stand out that are illustrative.

After it became known that I was able to hypnotize someone, there were frequent occasions when I was asked to give a demonstration. While gaining more experience I became especially intrigued by the regularity with which post-hypnotic suggestions were followed. In combination with my tendency to be somewhat mischievous, I was often drawn into doing things that appeared funny at the time (though now I look at it quite differently). One incident involved a fellow classmate in college who was particularly suggestable. This resulted in his being used as a subject on many occasions. He happened to live in a fraternity house, which had a number of rules as to when musical instruments could be played. Therefore it didn't take long for me to be giving him a post-hypnotic suggestion that he play his trumpet at four a.m. Sure enough at a little after four a.m. there he was playing away to the dismay of his fraternity brothers. He could give them no explanation other than to say he just felt impelled to do it.

The story of how this incident came about spread and a group approached me wanting to know if it was true. I explained what had happened, but they just didn't believe it was possible. One girl in particular scoffed at the idea and volunteered to be a subject so as to prove how nonsensical it was. As is so often the case she was, in fact, very receptive to moving into a hypnotic trance. I knew she was to attend a fraternity-sorority dinner that night, so after going through a variety of manuevers to show what can be done under hypnosis, I gave her a post-hypnotic suggestion. This was to clink her glass the moment a dessert plate was placed in front of her, after which to rise in order to sing a filthy song. That night the entire group (including myself) observed the event unseen in another room. The meal was completed, a dessert plate was put before her, and as expected she rose and clinked on her glass. The room became very quiet. Everyone's attention was focused upon her, wondering what announcement she was about to make. The tension increased as she remained silent, between what looked like attempts to speak. Each passing moment led to her blushing, trying once again, and then stopping. We, of course, knew what was happening and understood completely when she finally ran out of the room in extreme embarrassment. I felt terrible as the impact of her dilemma hit me (although I also couldn't help laughing at the same time). For the first time I saw the negative aspect of what I had been doing; up until then it had all seemed interesting and fun.

Nevertheless I did periodically continue, and in the process came in contact with some other people who were familiar with induction techniques. They were surprised to learn that I had never been hypnotized and invited me to be a subject. With some uneasiness I agreed. My experience was of going along with it, acting as though I was in a trance but fully aware of what was happening. Finally I just opened my eyes to announce what I had been doing only to have everyone laugh. They then began asking me questions as to whether I knew a variety of people by mentioning their names. Some sounded vaguely familiar though I couldn't place them, but then a name was spoken that really caught my attention. This was a child I knew very well from kindergarten, and had never seen since. To say I was amazed would be an understatement. They then explained how quickly I had gone under, so they brought me back to my kindergarten class where I proceeded to name each child. They then gave me a post-hypnotic suggestion that I would forget the entire scenario and believe I had been acting the entire time before waking me up. The force and power of this instrument that I had so casually been using really hit home, and my eyes were opening wider.

Not too long afterward I was visiting with a cousin who was staying next door to where I lived. The subject of hypnosis arose, with the people there being quite cynical about the reality of anything like that. She then coaxed me into showing them, for I was becoming reluctant to do so until I learned more about it. Against my better judgment I went ahead and the people watching were now seeing it for the first time. Any doubts they had quickly dissolved. Unbeknownst to me,in the middle of the night, my cousin awakened and was hysterical. Her arm, which I had used in inducing a trance was high up in the air and she just couldn't control it. Her roommates, not knowing what to do, had called the university health clinic. They, in turn, eventually got in touch with the head of the psychology department. Once he heard that I had hypnotized her earlier, he called me in to give me what was basically a lecture on the dangers I was flirting with. I did appreciate what he was saying and asked him a host of questions trying to understand more fully and not just take it as a prohibition.

Two nights later there was this now irate professor standing over my bed, as I was awakened from a deep sleep. He was furious as he threatened me with a long series of punishments if I did not immediately cease any kind of activity having to do with hypnosis. With that he stormed out of the room and left. Later I discovered that my cousin had once again been hysterical, apparently still reacting to her previous experience; again he was contacted, and this time came to see her. He took one look at her crying with her arm in the air, turned right around without saying a word and went directly to where I was. The incident was recorded in my file, and I received notice that I was being placed on probation. I just shrugged my shoulders and didn't really see any problem, for I had already decided to leave it alone at least until I had gained more knowledge.

Meanwhile my life went on without my giving any thought at all to my interest in hypnosis. It was as though I had outgrown whatever had fascinated me and was absorbed in other more important matters. I finished premed, entered medical school, got married, and developed new friends. Whatever hypnosis meant seemed to simply drop out of existence. All of this is a preamble to how it emerged once again, only now in response to a difficult situation. This time I was pleased with the consequences for the person I hypnotized, though it did pose some problems for me.

As was customary in an OB-gyne clerkship, two third year medical students were on call each night. On this particular evening it was a very good friend (fortunately) and myself who were scheduled. Much of the clinical staffs attention was focused on how to best manage what everyone could see was a tragic circumstance. The patient was a twelve year old blind girl who had been in hard labor for close to twenty-four hours when we arrived. Her cries of pain and terror with each contraction echoed throughout the halls. We found out the father was either her father or uncle, noone knew for sure, and we could just imagine what this whole experience must have been doing to her. Both of us had trouble understanding the casual, insensitive attitude of those responsible for her care, as well as why she was allowed to be in such hard labor for so long.

We were given abrupt answers for all of our questions, which were not at all satisfying. She was quite a sight to behold; tiny, a terrified look on her face, obviously exhausted, and every three minutes wailing in unbearable pain. All we were told was that they wanted to give her a chance to deliver naturally, since a caeserian section would leave a scar and perhaps affect her ability to deliver a child later in her life. It was now approaching thirty hours in labor and neither my friend nor I had any knowledge or experience to draw upon as to what the pros and cons were. Our continuing efforts to found out why they didn't just do a C section and get it over with, and even as to whether there wasn't some present danger to the baby and mother, were met with annoyance. We attended to her as well as we could, trying to reassure her or make some kind of contact that might be helpful. However, she was so enveloped with pain and terror there didn't seem to be any way to comfort her.

It was at this point that the idea of hypnotizing her arose within me. I told my friend what I had in mind and he looked at me like I must be nuts. We both knew it would do no good to ask for permission (the idea of things like that being a part of medicine was absolutely out of the question at that time). In addition if we did ask and got turned down, it would then be impossible to do. Having been in the service where you quickly learned to just do things like that, for in asking permission you only called attention to it, so we went ahead. He stood guard, so as to distract anyone from entering, while I was engaged in trying to hypnotize the blind girl. She was extraordinarily responsive, probably because she was so exhausted, and in a very short time was quietly resting. This in spite of the continuing frequent contractions. Various people then kept coming in to check on her, wondering what had happened. Their puzzlement was interesting to observe. She remained in a hypnotic trance, which became deeper with each repeated pelvic examination, for I had given her a post-hypnotic suggestion to that effect. At last they came to the conclusion that the baby was too large to deliver vaginally and went on to do a C-section.

Now came the time of reckoning, for there was much discussion as to the reason for the abrupt ending of her terrified cries. Many questions were asked to see if anyone had prescribed pain medication. At first they considered the possibility that she had just become too exhausted, until someone noticed a note in my file concerning my having been put on probation for being involved with hypnosis. When I was asked about it I answered honestly and then was called before a committee to present my side. This meeting did not last too long and for a time I was afraid it would result in some serious consequence, such as being expelled from school. I held my breath and hoped for the best.

After I described how and why I had done it, explaining why I didn't request permission, their questioning began. It centered upon my acting impulsively and upon my lack of knowledge in regard to obstetrics in general and the problem with this patient in particular. I openly admitted how little I knew, but called attention to my efforts to get some answers before I acted. I also wondered if they thought the experience was bad for the patient as I had tried to be sensitive to whether it was helpful. They had to admit that in this one situation it had been of some help, but they were worried that it might extend to others where it could be harmful. In that regard they then wanted me to assure them that I would never engage in such an action again. I could only say that I truly did not know if I would or wouldn't. However, I thought they were asking me the wrong question.

In my opinion the right question was whether I would not act, even if it was clear that my action could or would be helpful. Associated with that was my question to them. Now that they saw that what I did with this girl had a positive affect, would they be open to considering the same approach were it to come up again. Although they did not answer, the somewhat long silence that followed was a meaningful one. After this long pause, the head of the department quietly thanked me for coming and wished me luck in my career.

Following that incident I have had very little involvement with hypnosis. I have come to see it as mostly a negative procedure, for it is based upon creating an illusion, which can easily exploit human vulnerability. I am sure there are special circumstances where it might very well be useful, just as I believed it was with the twelve year old girl. Nevertheless, any procedure that depends upon deception and exploitation for its effectiveness must be suspect. The ease with which it can sometimes produce what appear to be spectacular results makes it quite seductive. It is for the same reason that quick fixes of any kind, cravings, and addictions are so easy to turn to as a solution to pain and discomfort. There is no question that the effects of hypnosis can be very powerful in the short run, making it tempting, while avoiding the hard work of genuine change in the long run. Looking back I can now see that for all the wrong reasons the OB-gyne group were right in their concern. Conversely, for many right reasons I was wrong in my conclusion.

The Last Chapter

It always makes me smile when I hear someone complain about the so-called fact that nothing has changed, or that everything remains the same. As far as I can see changes take place all of the time, both inside and outside of anyone I have ever known. Day into night; the seasons; conditions in which we live; moods; responses to hormonal changes; reactions to each other; the way the world is perceived; how we think and feel about ourselves to name only a few. Clearly these kinds of comments are both made and believed, so how is it possible for what is impossible to be believed and still be true? The only way I can conceive of it is by focusing one's attention exclusively upon one thing. Any given human being is so complex, and there is so much potentially available to be seen, that it is literally impossible to know it all in a lifetime. Yet it is not at all impossible to create the illusion that nothing is happening. How often have words been used to refer to someone as not living up to their potential. Of course that is true, since it is true of everyone. What it usually means, however, is that the person is not living up to or producing what someone else is expecting. I remember an eleven year old boy who was discussing with me what diagnosis he wanted me to put on an insurance form. We looked together at the myriad of labels, all of which carried a piece here or there that could conceivably be applied to him. Finally he looked up at me and with a confident tone in his voice said, "I know what my diagnosis is…. potentiosis!". He then went on to elaborate how everyone was always telling him that he wasn't living up to his potentials, and he heartily agreed because he could feel the truth in it(we did put it on the form under psychiatric condition, other: potentiosis. After some questioning the insurance co. accepted it).

As I come to the final chapter of this book, at a time when I am entering what could be thought of as the final chapter of my life(at least as I have known it thus far), the last chapter is a fitting title. I do know that I have learned alot over the years, to the point where I can see that I have barely scratched the surface of what my potential is for learning about myself(not to mention the overwhelming span of things to be learned in the world around me). I once saw a saying that expressed it succinctly, "It takes a long time to know nothing". In recent years my grandchildren, noting the evidence of my advancing age, will ask me when I am going to die. My answer to them sums up pretty well how I approach this aspect of my last chapter. I tell them that I consider the future unknowable, so I have no idea when or how. The one thing I do know at the moment is how I would like it to be. It is the final inning of a baseball game, with two outs and my team three runs behind. I come up to bat, hit a line drive between the outfielders, circle the bases using every ounce of energy that I can muster, and slide across home plate with the winning run as I move into wherever one goes in leaving this world. Most important is my desire to be awake and alert, so I have an opportunity to continue to learn as long as it is possible.

I once overheard two eight year old girls discussing a wide range of people they both knew. They were placing them into two categories, which they referred to as grown-ups and growing-ups. Upon listening closely I couldn't help but smile at the profound insight they displayed. Grown-ups thought they knew everything and were very rigid in their whole approach to life(especially in their inability to grant credibility to children). Growing—ups, on the other hand, were always open to learn something new and were fun to play with(in addition to paying close attention to what children had to contribute). The particular age of the individual had no relevance whatsoever as to which category they were placed into. In that context I am pleased to have reached my last chapter without becoming a grown-up.

My first recognition of having reached this phase of my life emerged as I neared my seventieth birthday. Up until that time birthdays had very little meaning to me, so I was puzzled when I found myself feeling excited about the prospect of celebrating this one. The day arrived before I had any words to explain my reaction. I woke up that morning with the words already formed in my head, which at first seemed a little silly. I thought, "well now I know what I want to be when I grow up!". Those words were saying that as I looked at myself, I liked what I saw. For years I had been told, usually in response to my acting upon one kind of idealistic principle or another, that I should just wait until I got older. Eventually I would see that, although I might be theoretically correct, a person simply cannot live that way in the "real" world. So there I was finally old enough, yet if anything I was even more idealistic. Much more important than that, however, was my acute awareness that I had alot more growing up to do.

Another key moment involved my entire family during the weeklong celebration of the fiftieth anniversary of our wedding. I first met my wife at a bowling alley, introduced by a close friend who sensed we would connect. He was certainly right in his assessment, though it took us both a while to realize just how deeply that link was forged, probably right from the beginning. First we had to learn about each other, more through body language and whatever else was communicated without words. I don't recall any serious discussions in those early days; it was mostly having fun in being together. Her honesty and naivete were refreshing to me, she was open to trying things that were unfamiliar to her, and I truly enjoyed her company. My first indication of something more serious welled up in me in response to seeing her play softball. Like so many other important things in my life it appears a little funny on the surface; but I thought, "wow, she throws like a guy!". Of course it reflected a shared interest in sports(so vital to me), but, in a way that I had no words for then, it was the potential for finding a friend and soulmate. The strength of our attachment became very apparent to us, and so we were married despite her family's concerted efforts to discourage her(they were worried, since I had no financial resources, and they thought of me as irresponsible from stories they had heard of my teenage years).

Well fifty years, four children, seven grandchildren, two step grandchildren, and a step great grandchild later, there we were celebrating the event in a setting that was just right for all of us—Hawaii! The way that decision was made symbolized for me the nature of our underlying friendship. We had both talked about visiting Hawaii someday all through the years. For one reason or another the time to go just didn't seem right; that is, until our fiftieth anniversary got close enough to feel real. We simply both immediately knew that was exactly the time and place where we wanted it to occur. The next question answered itself. Neither of us could picture the event without our children and grandchildren, so bingo everyone was notified over a year earlier to clear their schedule and off we would go. Happily it also clicked for all of the others old enough to have an opinion. Having lived a sufficient number of years to have attended many such events, it never made sense(to me at least)for the children to give the party to honor their parents. That seemed backwards, for as far as I could tell, my children had no choice in the matter. They had entered our lives to enrich it beyond anything I could have imagined, so they were the ones deserving to be honored.

The actual formal celebration took place on the last night and featured a planned ceremony, in which our original marital vows were replaced by what we would have said knowing what we do now. In our talking about it beforehand I knew I would speak spontaneously, but she felt it necessary to write her words down for fear she'd be left speechless. The moment came and I told her how convinced I was that I would never get married. On the one side every woman I had known or met seemed more concerned with how things looked rather than how they were, and on the other side I knew that I would be extremely difficult to live with. Trouble of one kind or another was always in the picture and I had no awareness then of how much I was drawn to it or created it in my attitude. I only knew that it woul;d be there. Amazingly to me I discovered that she loved that very quality in me, even though I often went too far. Furthermore she still laughed at my jokes. Thus I could sincerely offer her my devotion to the truth, my openness to talk about anything no matter what, and the depth to which I valued our friendship. In no way would I want us to form a committed relationship, only one wherein any problem could be met and solved by our strong desire to be genuine and honest. To me committments belong to jails and mental hospitals(and I'm not so sure about the latter), not human relationships. I believe obligations place one in chains, and I do not wish for either of us to be in that position. Finally I underscored my trust of her and my determination to be worthy of her trust.

Now it was her turn and she began by bringing to me what she knew I would treasure. She spoke from her heart without anything to read. She described what I had contributed to her life and the ways I had helped her to grow. She emphasized our many ups and downs, and how through it all she always felt a deep sense of trust. She agreed completely with how difficult a person I could be, but added that she had never been bored. Finally she joined me in placing her highest priority on nourishing our friendship, stressing that she too wanted nothing to do with obligations.. The evening ended with our looking around the room at the incredible blessing that we had been rewarded with. Each of the individuals we saw had a special significance, which enabled us to feel how much our love for each other had grown.

I have been told that a last chapter would not be complete without some kind of statement as to how I'd like to be remembered. No thoughts come to me about that,but if it boils down to how I like to be thought of right now it is easy to answer. More than anything else I like to be recognized for who and what I am!(warts and all). A powerful experience I had recently illustrates what it means to me when I am seen clearly. Many years ago I made a pact together with a best friend and soulmate. We trusted each other to look after the family left behind if and when the other left this world. Fortunately he lived long enough to see his children grow up, marry, and to enjoy his grandchildren(fortunately for them also to have experienced his influence). After he died I still felt bound to our pact, strengthened by my love for, and appreciation of, all of the members. Some I knew very well, some less well, but to all I am a symbolic carrier of the father and grandfather they have lost. Therefore it pleased me greatly when his thirteen year old grandson asked me to be a part of his upcoming bar mitzvah, because he wanted to feel his grandfather's presence. This was one family member I barely knew and I welcomed the opportunity .

The night before I was to be there I had a dream in which I entered a temple, only to see a man preparing to blow a shofar(ram's horn). Instead of the sound that I expected, what came out was bagpipe music. The dream made me laugh, since my soulmate was a true scotsman whose hobby was playing the bagpipes. I then felt totally prepared to bring him with me. The event began with a Friday night meal at a restaurant, followed by attending services at the temple. The moment I walked in I was greeted warmly by his parents and I told them my dream. They both gasped, and excitedly asked me to give a toast and tell everyone about my dream. They then explained that one of my friends sons wanted to play the bagpipes at the bar mitzvah, but the rabbi disapproved. In their eyes (and mine)what could be a more religious act than to honor their missing father and grandfather in this fashion. The fact that theirs was a mixed marriage meant nothing to him; the fact that his grandson was embracing a heartfelt spiritual ritual meant everything. So it was that I gave the toast, the rabbi reluctantly agreed to allow the bagpipes(though outside of the prayer room), and we were off to the temple.

Following the formal service(the bar mitzvah was to be the next day), dominated by the rabbi playing his guitar and singing as if to display his openness to flexibility in religious matters, he proceeded to conduct an interactive discussion about the meaning of God. It was quite an over intellectualized question and answer session, using concepts such as Godding(is God a verb instead of a noun)etc. I kept getting more annoyed as I listened, affected by the hypocrisy of his reaction to the bagpipes and self satisfied smile about his conduct of the service. When he then invited any further comments before closing, I decided to speak. I told him I was reminded of a group of Hebrew scholars huddled in a basement, feeling noble and righteous, as they nit picked various segments of the torah totally oblivious to the fact that God can only be seen and known through your heart. With that the service was ended. As I was leaving the wife of the bagpipe player (whom I am very fond of)whispered in my ear, "you're an inveterate iconoclast". I thought she was chastizing me for being an atheist(which was puzzling as she knew I was not). At any rate her words nagged at me, so I looked up iconoclast in the dictionary and smiled. It was right on. I am a person who attacks cherished beliefs and venerated institutions when they appear to me to be either erroneous or worse an outright sham.

Another example of how I am affected by others either misperceiving, or seeing me accurately, occurred quite a while ago when I decided to coach a boys baseball team. My decision was made after watching a game I loved destroyed by "well meaning" people trying to remove the ugly side of competitiveness from it. Providing this group of boys an experience of competition, which was highly rewarding for all of us, was great fun. We played teams from all over the city, and at the time were the only white team willing to play in black neighborhoods. It was a wonderful learning experience to come in contact with people from all walks of life. Our attitude also meant alot to some community leaders, who then invited us to participate in their annual tournament as an expression of their gratitude. The tournament took place in an area considered by some as potentially dangerous. I agreed and as the date came closer a few of the parents began to question me as to whether I would cancel it. With each passing day the questions changed to anxious demands that I look closely at the possible danger to their children. I tried everything I could think of to reassure them, for I knew the people involved, but my efforts were to no avail. Finally the night before, two of the parents confronted me angrily. They accused me of being reckless, unconcerned with the welfare of their children, and a dangerous influence upon them. I was therefore informed that two of the boys would not be allowed to participate. When I raised the question as to their racial bias, the attack only intensified. So it was that the tournament began without the two boys, while other parents even brought their younger children to watch in order to show their support. The following day everyone showed up including the two boys, and I was deeply touched when I discovered why. The two boys had gone to their parents and said with great emphasis, "what's the matter with you? Don't you know that he'd be dead before anything could happen to us?".

The boys had convinced their parents that they had complete confidence in me, which touched my heart when I heard about it. Here was a situation where both factors were at work; in one partial truths were woven into a fabric that was not me at all. My response was to primarily be concerned for the children who were exposed to such narrow, prejudicial attitudes. Basically, I shrugged my shoulders at how I was misunderstood. The boys recognized who and what I was, and the way that made me feel showed me that I really do care alot about being seen. The most accurate way to say it is that I care alot when it involves someone I care about. (I'm reminded of a very nosy person who persisted in asking me questions about myself, which I did not like. At one point he asked me why I was ignoring him. My answer said it all, "if I answered I wouldn't be ignoring you!"). It is especially meaningful to me when in being recognized it incorporates all of me. My grandson was talking to his father about me, advising him to ask me for my thoughts regarding a difficult situation he had trouble in figuring out how to handle. In his words, "I know he's very weird, so weird you never get his thoughts mixed up with yours, but sometimes he has really good ideas". These words were music to my ears(the root meaning of weird is to follow one's destiny).

Adding it all up I would say that I am alot of things, and I do like it when the whole package is recognized. I am an iconoclast, idealistic, at times foolish, often blind, passionate, devoted to the truth, furious about injustices, loyal, trustworthy(when I can see clearly), and definitely weird. I also notice a theme running through all of the important decisions I have made in my life; my choice of a mate, having a family, the profession I chose, and the role model I have embraced. The way I initially thought of them was characteristically short, to the point, yet at the same time obscure. Only later was I able to articulate the deeper meanings, which then brought clarity to why I followed the directions they pointed toward. The choice of a mate, because she was honest and could throw like a guy; having a family, so I'd have someone to talk to; the profession I selected from seeing the movie"Spellbound"; and my role model, Mr. Magoo. It's really not such a mystery. Throwing like a guy meant able to value someone who would both say and take things like they really are, with a willingness and desire to develop that same attribute(in addition to loving sports). Having someone to talk to meant that infants and children speak a language I love: straight, not dependent solely on words, and often highly symbolic. In short I can know them and they in turn can know me, with the emphasis being on whatever is true. The movie portrayed that same message, except this time in searching for a hidden truth. In regard to Mr. Magoo, his image presents a picture of not seeing the truth(or anything else for that matter)in a benign and humorous fashion. Therefore this caricature serves as a friendly reminder to me, always more effective than something harsh or punitive, which my playful attitude has accepted as a role model.

I was once asked what I thought I would do if I was rendered completely helpless by some paralyzing illness. What popped out was that I would be a poet. It made me laugh, though I knew I was serious, because of all the things that I have shown any talent for, or even interest in, this would be far down the list. The only thing that came close was my love of limericks, which can hardly be considered to be poetry in the usual sense of the word. However, not too long ago, I had a dream in which I recited a poem. Upon awakening I quickly wrote it down before it could fade away into oblivion. At this moment it seems a fitting way to close this book.

The Dream

There's a sentry at the gates of Hell
So mark the spot; it's served you well
An angel dressed in fiery clothes
To guard the choices you'd oppose
The pain it's caused makes thanks come slow
A sore spot touched is a crushing blow
Rough edges block the need to swallow
Yet to get what's yours lets good things follow
A warrior holds a powerful sword
To use it well is life's reward
Though it took many years to find
And I mourn what's left in being blind
I'm pleased I continue to muddle through
Oh how I love old Mr. Magoo
There are reasons when I cannot see
They must be honored for me to be me

978-0-595-35717-8
0-595-35717-2

www.ingramcontent.com/pod-product-compliance
Lightning Source LLC
Chambersburg PA
CBHW051449280526
45785CB00003B/1485